Introduction to Computed Tomography

INTRODUCTION TO COMPUTED TOMOGRAPHY

Lois E. Romans, R.T.
CT Technologist
Botsford General Hospital
Farmington Hills, Michigan
President
Enterprises for Continuing Education, Inc.
Brighton, Michigan

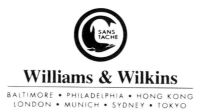

Williams & Wilkins

BALTIMORE • PHILADELPHIA • HONG KONG
LONDON • MUNICH • SYDNEY • TOKYO

A WAVERLY COMPANY

1995

Acquisitions Editor: Elizabeth A. Nieginski
Project Editor: Amy G. Dinkel
Production Coordinator: Peter J. Carley
Illustrator: Patricia MacAllen

Copyright © 1995
Williams & Wilkins
Suite 5025
Rose Tree Corporate Center
Building Two
1400 North Providence Road
Media, PA 19063-2043

Library of Congress Cataloging-in-Publication Data

Romans, Lois E.
    Introduction to computed tomography / Lois E. Romans.
        p.   cm.
    Includes bibliographical references and index.
    ISBN 0-683-07353-2
    1. Tomography.   I. Title.
    [DNLM: 1. Tomography, X-Ray Computed.   WN 160 R759i 1995]
RC78.7.T6R66   1995
616.07'572--dc20
DNLM/DLC
for Library of Congress   94-43673
                                                                  CIP

Printed in the United States of America

Library of Congress Cataloging in Publication Data

                                            95   96   97   98
                            1   2   3   4   5   6   7   8   9   10

Dedication

This book is dedicated to my husband, Ken, and my daughters, Ashleigh, Chelsea, and Abigail.

Contributor

James A. Tomlinson, M.S.
Diagnostic Radiological Physicist
Diplomate
American Board of Radiology
Vice President
Medical Physics Consultants, Inc.
Ann Arbor, Michigan

Contents

Foreword   xi

Acknowledgments   xiii

Section I   Computed Tomography Concepts

1   Basic Principles of Computed Tomography   3

2   Creating the Computed Tomography Image   8

3   Factors Affecting Image Quality   19

4   Methods of Data Acquisition   24

5   Image Display   33

6   Radiation Dosimetry   43

7   Enhancement Techniques   51

8   General Imaging Techniques   60

Section II   Examination Protocols

9   Head and Brain   71

10   Neck   77

11   Chest   79

12   Abdomen   81

13   Pelvis   85

14   Spine   86

15   Musculoskeletal System   90

16   Specialized CT Studies   91

17   Interventional CT   96

Appendices   98

Glossary   100

Bibliography   104

Index   105

Foreword

The word tomography has as its root, *tomo,* which means "to cut." In the case of computed tomography, or CT as it is often abbreviated, a sophisticated computerized method is used to obtain data and transform them into "cuts," or cross-sectional slices of the human body.

The first scanners were limited in the ways in which these cuts could be performed. All early scanners produced axial cuts; that is, slices looked like the rings of a tree visualized in the cut edge of a log. Therefore, it was common to refer to older scanning systems as computerized axial tomography, hence the common acronym, CAT scan.

Newer model scanners offer options in more than just the transverse plane. Therefore, the word "axial" has been dropped from the name of current CT systems. If the old acronym CAT is used, it now represents the words computer *assisted* tomography.

The purpose of this text is to take the complicated technical process of CT scanning and break it down into digestible components that can be more easily understood. My philosophy can be summed up in the phrase, "You don't have to know how to build a car to be a good driver." This book provides only the technical detail essential to understanding the modality. It is designed for the technologist, resident, or medical salesperson who wishes to understand the process without having to sift through highly technical information that has little bearing on the actual outcome of scanning. It *is* a fascinating modality, and I hope that the basics provided here will encourage many students to continue on to more advanced study.

Identifying cross-sectional anatomy is essential to the art of CT scanning, but is beyond the scope of this text. The understanding and identification of cross-sectional anatomy are best dealt with in a text devoted to that subject and written by a physician. Therefore, anatomy is only described in this text when it directly impacts the scanning protocol, and even in these cases is only superficially covered.

Included in the text is a chapter on radiation dosimetry written by a radiation physicist. I've found that nearly everyone working in the field—radiologist, technologist, and manufacturer's representatives alike—are sorely lacking in their understanding of the radiation dose delivered to the patient. To make informed choices for our patients, learning elementary CT dosimetry is essential. Jim Tomlinson has done a wonderful job of explaining the basics in language that is understandable to us non-physicists.

A section outlining common scanning protocols is included in the second section of the book. These protocols are intended to be general guidelines and may be helpful to a department that has just purchased its first CT system. It will also help the practicing technologist by providing the "norm" among departments across the country. In addition, the rationale behind many of the variations in scan procedure is explained.

As the field of computed tomography continues to evolve, it becomes even more important that the basic principles be understood. Only with this foundation can we hope to comprehend the many new developments that face us as we head into a new century of medicine.

Acknowledgments

Special thanks to Dr. Andrew Mizzi from Botsford General Hospital for his help in editing the medical chapters. I would like to acknowledge the great expertise of Dr. Stan Fox with General Electric Medical Systems and Jim Tomlinson of Medical Physics Consultants. Their help in the area of physics was invaluable. Two fellow technologists, Renee Maas and Carolyn Miller, deserve special thanks for reviewing each chapter as it was written and helping me keep the focus of the text simple and practical. I would also like to thank Dr. David Wiseley of Botsford Hospital for his patience in sharing his considerable knowledge with me. Finally, I would like to thank Dr. David Yates of Oakwood Hospital, my first teacher in CT, for his enthusiasm and encouragement.

Section I

COMPUTED TOMOGRAPHY CONCEPTS

Chapter 1

BASIC PRINCIPLES OF COMPUTED TOMOGRAPHY

TERMINOLOGY

The process by which computed tomography (CT) evolved could fill a volume in itself. However, for the sake of simplicity, only a few key elements will be mentioned.

Although all CT manufacturers begin with the same basic form, each attempts to improve the technology and add features to set their scanner apart in the marketplace. As each new feature is added to a system, it is given a name by the manufacturer. For this reason, the same feature may have a variety of different names, depending on the manufacturer.

For example, the preliminary image each scanner produces has many names. Siemens refers to this image as a topogram; General Electric calls it a scout; Toshiba calls it a scanogram; and the list goes on.

One of the most recent and dramatic developments in the field, **continuous acquisition scanning,** provides an example of the variation in names. Siemens was the first company to market this product. Under the label of **spiral scanning,** Siemens attempted to capitalize on their advantage. Siemens marketing referred to spiral scanning as the wave of the future and insisted that it was essential to modern scanning. To a large degree, this strategy was successful.

Siemens' primary competitor, General Electric, made the decision not to release their continuous acquisition scanner until certain flaws were worked out. They ultimately produced a scanner that overcame some of the disadvantages inherent in the Siemens' initial spiral system. However, General Electric lost precious time and market share in the 2-year interim. How could they regain their place in the market? How could they convince customers that they truly had a different (and, in their opinion, superior) system? To show customers that their continuous acquisition scanner required serious attention and was not merely a copy of the Siemens scanner,

General Electric marketed their option as **helical scanning.** Therefore, when comparing spiral and helical scanning, it is important to understand that both accomplish the same goal with the same basic technology; however, each has its own emphasis, with corresponding strengths and weaknesses.

Comparing CT systems from different manufacturers is a difficult task. Manufacturers mix a fair amount of marketing strategy in with facts. Often, equipment specifications and statistics are skewed to conceal a system's deficiencies. Rather than acknowledge a shortcoming within their system, many companies insist that a feature is not necessary. The best way for any professional to make an accurate assessment of a specific system's strengths and weaknesses is to understand completely the basic principles involved in CT. Equipped with this understanding, it is much easier to comprehend innovations and to sort facts from marketing claims.

These inconsistencies add to a beginner's confusion. Although standardization of terms is frequently discussed among technologists and radiologists, it is unlikely to be achieved. The market forces that created the present system are strong. A table (see Appendix A) is included to reduce potential confusion created by inconsistent terminology. The major manufacturers are listed, followed by the designation that each gives each CT function. Each function is described in a generic way.

This text refers to each function by the name that best describes it or by the term that is most widely used. Once the student learns what each operation accomplishes, switching terms to accommodate scanners is easy.

CT DEFINED

CT uses a computer to process information collected from the passage of x-ray beams through an area of anatomy. The images created are cross-sectional. To help the novice to visualize CT, the often-used loaf of bread

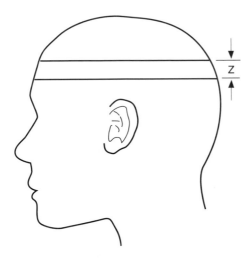

Fig. 1–1. Z axis.

analogy is useful. If the patient's body is imagined to be a loaf of bread, each CT slice correlates to a slice of the bread. The crust of the bread is analogous to the skin of the patient's body, and the white portion of bread relates to the patient's internal organs.

The individual CT slice shows only the parts of the anatomy imaged at that level. Therefore, a scan taken at the level of the sternum would show portions of lung, mediastinum, and ribs, but would not show portions

of, for example, kidneys and bladder. It is essential to have a firm knowledge of anatomy. It is equally important to identify the location of each organ relative to the others.

Each CT slice represents a specific plane in the patient's body. The thickness of the plane is referred to as its **Z axis.** The Z axis determines the thickness of the slices (see Figure 1–1). The operator selects the thickness of the slice from choices available on the specific scanner. Selecting a slice thickness limits the x-ray beam so that it passes only through this volume. Hence, scatter radiation and superimposition of other structures are greatly diminished. The data that form the CT slice are further sectioned into elements: width is indicated by x, and height is indicated by y, as seen in Figure 1–2. Each one of these two-dimensional squares is a **pixel** (picture element) displayed on the CT monitor (see Figure 1–3). The CT image is a composite of pixels for each slice. If the Z axis is taken into account, the result is a cube, rather than a square. This cube is referred to as a **voxel** (volume element). A **matrix** is the grid formed from the rows and columns of pixels. Although some new scanners have a matrix size of 1024, the most common matrix size is 512. This size translates to 512 rows of pixels down and 512 columns of pixels across. The total number of pixels present in a matrix is

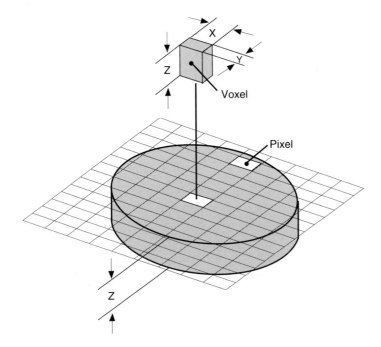

Fig. 1–2. The gray disc represents a cross-sectional slice corresponding to the patient. To create an image, the patient's data are segmented. A pixel is a two-dimensional square. A voxel incorporates the thickness of the slice, and is a three-dimensional cube.

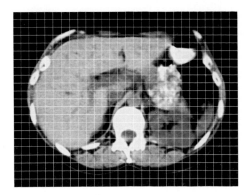

Fig. 1–3. The computed tomographic (CT) image is a composite of pixels, which are two-dimensional squares displayed on the CT monitor.

the product of the number of rows and the number of columns, in this case 512 × 512 (262,144). Each pixel contains information that the computer obtains from scanning.

BEAM ATTENUATION

The structures in a CT image are represented by varying shades of gray. The creation of these shades of gray is based on basic radiation principles. X-ray energy passes through or is stopped by a given structure in varying amounts, depending on the density of the structure. This phenomenon is referred to as **attenuation** of the x-ray beam.

In conventional radiography, the x-ray beam passes through the patient's body and exposes the photographic film. Similarly, in CT, the x-ray beam passes through the patient's body and is recorded by detectors. The

computer processes this information to form the CT image. The quantity of x-ray beams that pass through the body determines the shades of gray on the image in both cases.

By convention, x-ray beams that pass through objects unimpeded are represented by a black area on the image. Conversely, x-ray beams that are completely stopped by an object cannot be detected; therefore, the place on the image where the beam is halted is white. All intermediate attenuations are represented by various shades of gray.

As stated, the density of an object determines how much of the x-ray beam passes through the object, but what exactly is density?

The density of an object is determined by its molecular structure. Elements with a higher atomic number have more circulating electrons and heavier nuclei. The more atomic particles there are in an element, the more tightly packed that molecular structure is. In turn, the element is denser.

Metals are generally quite dense and have the greatest capacity for beam attenuation. Surgical clips and other metallic objects consequently are represented on the CT image as white areas. Air (gas) has very low density, so it has little attenuation capacity. Air-filled structures (e.g., lungs) are represented on the CT image as black areas.

Oral or intravenous administration of a contrast agent fills the structure with a higher-density material, which increases the structure's beam attenuation. The structure is highlighted on the CT image. Figure 1–4A shows an image taken at the level of the liver

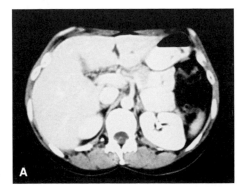

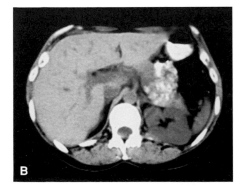

Fig. 1–4. (A) Slice of the liver taken without intravenous contrast enhancement. Note the low attenuation of the blood vessels and left kidney. (B) Slice taken after the administration of intravenous contrast media.

without intravenous contrast enhancement. Figure 1–4B shows the same slice after the injection of an iodinated contrast medium. The blood vessels arc highlighted because of their increased density.

It is important to remember that a contrast agent does not permanently change the physical properties of the structure containing it. A helpful analogy may be that of a glass of water viewed from a distance. Because the water is clear, it is difficult to see the outline of the glass clearly. If coloring is added to the water, the outline of the glass becomes much more visible. The actual glass is not changed; when the colored water is replaced by clear water, the glass reverts to its former appearance.

Hounsfield Units

The degree of beam attenuation on a CT image can be quantified. Measurements are expressed in **Hounsfield units** (HUs), named after Godfrey Newbold Hounsfield, who pioneered CT development. These units are also referred to as **CT numbers.**

Hounsfield arbitrarily assigned water the number 0 (Figure 1–5). He assigned the number 1000 to bone and −1000 to air. Objects with a beam attenuation less than that of water have an associated negative number. Conversely, substances with an attenuation greater than that of water have a proportionally positive Hounsfield unit.

With this system, a measurement of an unknown structure that appears on an image is taken and compared with measurements of known substances. It is then possible to approximate the composition of the unknown structure.

For example, a slice of abdomen shows a circular low-attenuation (dark) area on the left kidney. By taking a Hounsfield reading of this area, it is discovered to measure 4 HU. It can then be assumed that it is a fluid-filled mass (most likely a cyst). It is important to keep in mind that the reading for the assumed cyst is not exact. In this example, it is suspected that the mass is fluid because its measurement is close to that of pure water. The difference of 4 units could be caused by impurities in the cyst (it is not likely that a cyst would consist of pure water). Other factors that contribute to an inaccurate Hounsfield measurement are discussed later in the text (see Chapter 2).

It is considered standard procedure at many institutions to include a Hounsfield measurement on specific images. Each scanning procedure in which this practice is commonly expected is notated in the following chapters. Chapter 5 describes measurement systems available with CT.

Not all radiologists agree on the importance and accuracy of the Hounsfield unit in CT. Although many would not make a diagnosis without first obtaining a measurement, there are others who believe that the inclusion of too many factors can cause inaccurate measurements. Some of the factors that affect measurement accuracy are volume averaging and artifacts. Artifacts and their causes are discussed in Chapter 3.

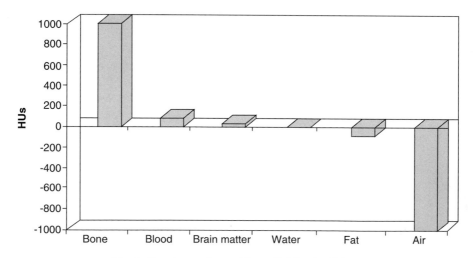

Fig. 1–5. Approximate Hounsfield units (HUs).

Volume Averaging

All CT examinations are performed by obtaining a series of slices through a designated area of interest. The nature of the anatomy and the pathology suspected determine how the examination is performed. Scanners allow the technologist to select slice thickness, and scanners vary in the thickness choices available.

In general, the smaller the object being scanned, the thinner the CT slice required. Again, the loaf of bread analogy is helpful. This time, it is raisin bread. As the loaf is sliced and examined, it is found that some slices contain raisins and others do not. If the slices are thick, it increases the possibility that even though a given slice contains a raisin, it will be obscured by the bread. If the slices are thin, the likelihood of missing a raisin decreases, but the total number of slices increases. If the analogy is switched to rye bread, and caraway seeds are being sought, it is easy to understand how the slice thickness must be adjusted depending on the object being examined.

Thicker CT slices increase the likelihood of missing very small areas. For example, if 10-mm slices are made, and the area of pathology measures just 2 mm, normal tissue represents 8 mm and is averaged in with the pathologic tissue, in a fashion similar to the raisins in the bread. This process is referred to as **volume averaging,** or **partial volume effect.** Therefore, if an area is suspicious for a mass, but not definitive, scanning the same area at a thinner slice may be useful.

Why do some scanning protocols use thicker cuts? Although 1-mm or 2-mm slice thicknesses are available on most scanners, the routine use of such thin slices is not practical. Done at 2-mm slices, a routine abdominal scan would require more than 150 slices, which would deliver an unacceptably large radiation dose to the patient. Scanning procedures are designed to provide the best mix of lesion detection and acceptable dose. It is important to understand, however, that no protocol is correct for every patient. The technologist, with input from a radiologist if necessary, must adjust the examination to meet the needs of the individual patient.

CHAPTER SUMMARY

A variety of names describe the same basic CT function, dependent on the manufacturer. Images produced in CT are cross-sectional. The CT image is made up of many small squares called pixels. All of the pixels together form a matrix. If the thickness of the slice is considered, then the elements are called voxels. The plane that refers to the thickness of a slice is the Z axis.

CT is based on attenuation of the x-ray beam as it passes through a specific plane of anatomy. Beam attenuation is dependent on the density of the object that the x-ray beam passes through. Beam attenuation is quantified by Hounsfield units. These units are not absolute because their accuracy may be compromised. Volume averaging occurs when different tissues are averaged together. This process distorts CT measurements. This phenomenon is also called partial volume effect.

REVIEW QUESTIONS

1. What defines the Z axis?
2. Define pixel, voxel, and matrix.
3. Define beam attenuation. What determines a structure's ability to attenuate the x-ray beam?
4. What does an intravenous or oral contrast agent do to an organ's attenuation capability?
5. What unit quantifies a structure's ability to attenuate the x-ray beam?
6. Why might a 2-mm lesion go undetected if a 10-mm slice thickness is used?

Chapter 2

CREATING THE COMPUTED TOMOGRAPHY IMAGE

Scanners vary widely in their mechanical makeup. The ideal configuration and composition of detectors and tube are debated topics within the industry. Each manufacturer claims that its scanner design is the best. Unfortunately, it is impossible to state unequivocally which set of design factors produces the best overall CT scanner. It is not essential to understand the precise makeup of every scanner available on the market to perform high-quality studies. This chapter provides a basic understanding of CT image production.

OVERVIEW OF CT OPERATION

The components that produce x-ray beams are housed in the gantry. The x-ray tube contains filaments that provide the electrons that create x-ray beams. This is accomplished by heating the filament until electrons start to boil off and break away from the filament. The generator produces high voltage or kV and transmits it to the x-ray tube. This high voltage propels the electrons from the x-ray tube filament to the anode. The quantity of electrons propelled is referred to as tube current and is measured in one thousandth of an ampere, which is referred to as milliamperes (mA). The electrons then strike the rotating anode target and disarrange the electrons in the target material. The result is the production of heat and x-ray photons. In an effort to spread the heat over a larger area, the target rotates. Increasing the voltage increases the energy with which the electrons strike the target and the intensity of the x-ray beam.

The ability of the tube to withstand the resultant heat is called its **heat capacity.** The ability of the tube to rid itself of the heat is referred to as its **heat dissipation.** The length and frequency of scans are determined in part by the tube's heat capacity and dissipation rate.

The x-ray beams that pass through the patient strike the detector. If the detector is made from a solid-state scintillator material, the energy of the x-ray beams stopped will be turned into light. Other elements in the detector, usually a photodiode, convert the light levels into an electric current. If the detector is of the xenon gas variety, the striking photon ionizes the xenon gas. These ions are accelerated by the high voltage on the detector plates.

Regardless of the detector material, each detector cell is sampled many times, as many as 1000 times per second, by the data acquisition system (DAS). Analog-to-digital converters in the DAS are used to convert the electric signal to a digital format. Each complete sample is called a view. The digital data from the DAS are then transmitted to the central processing unit (CPU). The CPU is often referred to as the brain of the CT scanner.

The reconstruction processor is often an array processor with multiple parallel channels that takes the individual views and reconstructs the densities within the slice. To create an image, information from the DAS must be translated into a matrix. To do so, the system assigns each pixel in the matrix one value or density number. This density number, or Hounsfield unit (HU), is the average of all measurements for that pixel. These digitized data are then sent to a display processor that converts them into television shades of gray. The resulting image is then displayed on the cathode-ray tube (CRT) monitor.

Although there is wide variation in the design of scanners, there are some characteristics that they share. The CT process can be broken down into three segments: data acquisition, image reconstruction, and image display. This chapter discusses the data acquisition and image reconstruction aspects of image formation. Displaying the image is discussed in Chapter 5.

DATA ACQUISITION

The components that are involved in this phase of image creation are the generator, the gantry, and the patient table.

Generator

The generator produces high voltage and transmits it to the x-ray tube. The power capacity of the generator is listed in kilowatts (kW). A generator can have a single kilovolt-peak (kVp) or variable kVp output. Accuracy is more easily achieved in single kVp systems. However, variable kVp systems allow for an increased capacity to discriminate between different tissues. A sophisticated generator is necessary to produce accurate output with a variable kVp system.

Gantry

The **gantry** is the part of the CT system that laymen fondly refer to as "the big doughnut." Gantries vary in total size as well as in the diameter of the opening. The gantry houses the x-ray tube, which moves in a circular path within it. X-ray energy is emitted as the tube travels along this path to reach the patient, who is placed within the opening. Some of the x-ray energy passes through the patient, and some is attenuated or scattered. The x-ray beams that pass through the patient are retrieved by the computer detectors.

Scanner Generation

The configuration of the x-ray tube to the detectors determines scanner generation. The first system produced by the now defunct EMI medical division had a design that is referred to as first generation. A thin x-ray beam passed linearly over the patient, and a single detector followed on the opposite side of the patient. The tube and detector were then rotated slightly, and the process was repeated until a 180° arc was covered. Scan times were very long. This design is no longer in use.

As new developments in scanning occurred, each new tube–detector design was referred to by a consecutive generation number. The second-generation design is one in which the x-ray beam also passed linearly across the patient before rotating. However, a fan-shaped x-ray beam was used, rather than the thin beam used with first-generation designs. Only part of the field of view could be covered with this fan beam. A detector array was also incorporated in the second-generation design. While scan times were shorter than in the original design, they were still very long. This type of design is also no longer used.

The next advance in CT technology brought the third-generation design. This design consists of a detector array and an x-ray tube that produces a fan-shaped beam that covered the entire field of view and a detector array. It was no longer necessary to translate the beam and detector as both could move in a circle within the gantry. The rotating detector design allows all of the readings that make up a view to be recorded instantaneously and simultaneously. This greatly reduced scan times. These are sometimes referred to as rotate–rotate scanners. The third-generation design is the most widely used configuration in the industry today (see Figure 2–1).

Fourth-generation scanners use a detector array that is fixed in a 360° circle within the gantry. The tube rotates within the fixed detector array and produces a fan-shaped beam. However, the number of detectors in use at any one time is controlled by the width of the beam. In the stationary detector design, the readings that make up a view are recorded consecutively over approximately one-fifth of the scan time. Fourth-generation scanners are also called rotate-only systems. Picker is the only company currently using the fourth-generation design (see Figure 2–2).

Variations of these basic designs have been introduced and then abandoned. The only other design currently in use is called **electron beam imaging.** It differs from conventional CT in a number of ways. This system, which was originally produced by Imatron, uses a large electron gun as its x-ray beam source. A massive anode target is placed in a semicircular ring around the patient. Neither the x-ray beam source nor the detectors move, and the scans can be acquired in a short time. Because of its many fundamental differences from conventional CT, electron beam imaging is not discussed in this text.

X-ray Beam Source

X-ray tubes produce the x-ray energy that creates the CT image. Their design is a modification of a standard rotating anode tube, such as the type used in angiography. An enormous amount of stress is placed on the CT tube. Scanning protocols require multiple exposures in a short time, performed on numerous patients per day. Table 2–1 compares the typical daily number of exposures in a busy department for standard radiography, angiography, and CT. It is easy to see why a CT tube

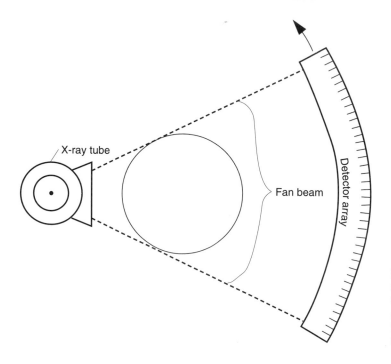

Fig. 2–1. A third-generation scanner design is one in which the x-ray tube is placed opposite the detector array. Both the tube and the detector move in a circle within the gantry.

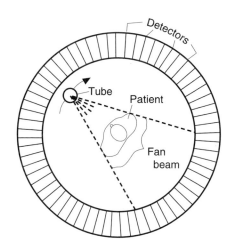

Fig. 2–2. A fourth-generation scanner design uses a detector array that is fixed in a 360° circle within the gantry. The tube rotates within the gantry.

Table 2–1. Comparison of Typical Number of Exposures in an 8-hour Day

Standard Radiography	Angiography	CT
75 exposures	60 exposures	960 exposures

must be designed to handle such stress. The way a tube dissipates the heat that is created during the production of an x-ray beam is critical. All manufacturers list generator and tube cooling capabilities in their product specifications. These specifications usually list the system generator's maximum power. Generator power is listed in kilowatts (kW). Also listed is the anode heat capacity [in million heat units (MHU)] and the maximum anode heat dissipation rate [in thousand heat units (KHU)]. These specifications can be helpful in comparing various CT systems. It is important to remember that these values represent the upper limit of tube performance. It is also important to compare the length of protocols that the tube will allow and how quickly they can be repeated.

All x-ray beam sources for CT and conventional radiography produce x-ray energy that is polychromatic. The x-ray beams emitted are over a broad spectrum of energies. Some of the x-ray photons are weak, and others are relatively strong. It is essential to understand how this basic property affects the image. Low-energy x-ray beams are more readily attenuated by the patient. The detectors cannot differentiate and adjust for differences in attenuation that are caused by low-energy x-ray beams. To the detectors, any x-ray beam that reaches the detector is treated identically, whether it began with high or low energy. This phenomenon can produce artifacts. **Artifacts** are objects seen on the image but not present in the object scanned. Artifacts always degrade the image. Artifacts that result from preferential absorption of the low-energy photons, leaving higher-intensity photons to strike the detector array, are called **beam hardening artifacts.** The overall result is a general decrease in the CT numbers. This effect is the most obvious when the x-ray beam must first penetrate a dense structure, such as at the base of the skull. This artifact is seen as dark streaks across the images. Beam hardening is also seen as vague areas of decreased density and cupping artifacts (see Figure 2–3).

Filtering the x-ray beam with a substance such as Teflon or aluminum helps to reduce the range of x-ray energies that reach the patient. Creating a more uniform beam intensity improves the CT image by reducing artifacts. These mechanical filters shape the x-ray beam intensity. Filtering removes soft, or low-energy, x-ray beams and minimizes patient exposure.

Certain filters are used to reduce the beam intensity at the periphery of the beam, corresponding to the thinner areas of a patient's anatomy. Filtering produces a smaller degree of photon intensity. Because of their shape, they are often referred to as **bow tie filters.** (see Figure 2 4). There are also software corrections that can be made after the x-ray beams are attenuated by the patient, reducing the effect of beam hardening on the image.

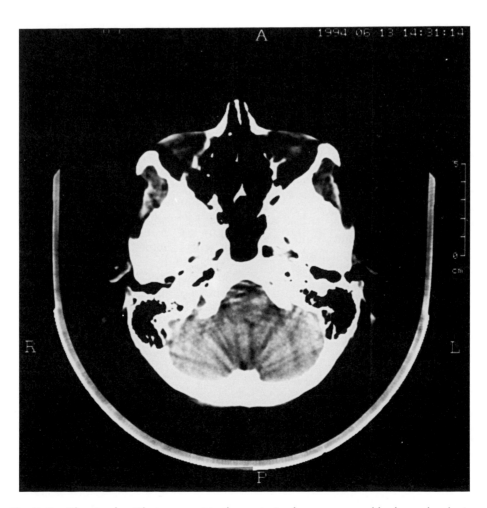

Fig. 2–3.   The streak artifacts present in the posterior fossa are caused by beam hardening.

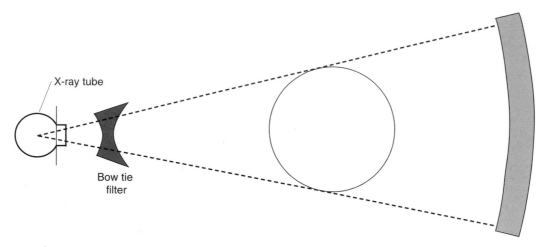

Fig. 2–4. Filtering shapes the x-ray beam intensity. Removing low-energy x-rays minimizes patient exposure and produces a more uniform beam.

Collimation

The source collimators are located in the x-ray tube and limit the amount of x-ray beam emerging to thin ribbons of 1 to 10 mm. They resemble small shutters with an opening that adjusts, dependent on the operator's selection of slice thickness. The advantage of this fine collimation is the reduction of scatter radiation. Scatter radiation reduces image quality and increases the radiation dose to the patient. Reducing the scatter improves contrast resolution. **Contrast resolution** is the ability to differentiate small density differences on the image.

The source collimator controls the slice thickness by narrowing or widening the x-ray beam. Scanners vary in the choices of slice thickness available. Choices range from 1 to 10 mm.

Detectors

Detectors can be made from different substances with their own advantages and disadvantages. The optimal characteristics of a detector are: (1) high detector efficiency, defined as the ability of the detector to capture transmitted photons and change them to electronic signals; (2) low afterglow, defined as a brief, persistent flash of scintillation that must be taken into account and subtracted before image reconstruction; (3) high scatter suppression; and (4) high stability. Overall detector efficiency is the product of a number of factors. These are: (a) stopping power of the detector material; (b) scintillator efficiency [in solid state types]; (c) charge collection efficiency [in xenon types]; (d) geometric efficiency, defined as the amount of space occupied by the detector collimator plates relative to the surface area of the detector; and (e) scatter rejection.

Detectors currently in use are made of either xenon gas or solid-state crystals (see Table 2–2). Pressurized xenon gas fills hollow chambers to produce detectors that absorb approximately 60% to 87% of the photons that reach them. Xenon gas detectors are significantly less expensive to produce, somewhat easier to calibrate, and highly stable.

A xenon detector channel consists of three tungsten plates. When a photon enters the channel, it ionizes the xenon gas. These ions are accelerated and amplified by the electric

Table 2–2. Characteristics of Detectors

Solid-State Crystal	Pressurized Xenon Gas
High photon absorption	Moderate photon absorption
Sensitive to temperature, moisture	Highly stable
Solid material	Low-density material (gas)
Can exhibit afterglow	No afterglow
No front window loss	Losses due to front window and the space taken up by plates

field between the plates. The collected charge produces an electric current. This current is then processed as raw data. A disadvantage of xenon gas is that it must be kept under pressure in an aluminum casing. This casing filters the x-ray beam to a certain extent. Loss of x-ray beams in the casing window and the space taken up by the plates are the major factors hampering detector efficiency.

Solid-state crystal detectors are made from a variety of materials, including sodium iodide, bismuth germinate, cadmium tungstate, cesium iodide, and ceramic rare earth. They absorb nearly 100% of photons that reach them. In addition, there is no loss in the front window, as in xenon systems. This increased absorption efficiency is the chief advantage of solid-state detectors. Solid-state detectors may produce a brief afterglow. However, new solid-state detectors reduce or eliminate this disadvantage. This type of detector is more sensitive to fluctuations in temperature and moisture than the gas variety.

When an x-ray beam strikes a solid-state detector, it is absorbed by the scintillator material in the detector. This material then generates a corresponding level of light. The detector converts the light levels into an electric current, which is then processed as raw data.

The relative placement of the detectors affects the amount of scatter radiation that reaches the image. Figure 2–5 shows the relation between detector arrangement and scatter acceptance.

Patient Table

The patient lies on the table and is moved within the gantry for scanning. The process of moving the table by a specified measure is most commonly called **incrementation,** but is also referred to as **feed, step,** or **index.**

A numeric readout of the table location relative to the gantry is displayed. When the patient is placed within the gantry, an anatomic landmark, such as the xiphoid or the iliac crest, is adjusted so that it lies at the scan point. At this level, the table is **referenced,** which means that the table position is manually set at zero by the technologist. Accurate table referencing helps to maintain consistency between examinations. For example, if a lesion is seen on an image that is 50 mm

inferior* to the xiphoid landmark (zero point), the patient is removed from the gantry, and a ruler is used to measure 50 mm inferior from the xiphoid. This point provides an approximation of the location of the lesion. This system is also helpful if the scan will be repeated at a later date, exclusively through the area of interest. For this reason, the setting of landmarks must be consistent among CT staff.

The specifications of tables vary, but all have certain weight restrictions. If the patient's weight exceeds the specified limits, scanning is often still possible. However, the table increments may not be as accurate. This problem affects small table increments more than those larger than 5 mm. On most scanners, it is possible to place the patient either head first or feet first, supine or prone. Patient position within the gantry depends on the examination being performed.

IMAGE RECONSTRUCTION

As the x-ray tube travels along its circular path, continuous x-ray energy is being generated. The path that the x-ray beam takes from the tube to the detector is referred to as a **ray.** The detector reads each arriving ray and measures how much of the beam is attenuated. This measurement is called a **ray sum.** A complete set of ray sums is known as a **view.** A view is similar to a person looking at an object. From only one angle, it is difficult to obtain a true understanding of the shape of the object. To obtain the most realistic picture of the object, it would be best to walk around and observe it from many angles. The observer's final evaluation of the object would involve all of his observations. The CT image is created in much the same way. Many views are needed to create an image.

The system accounts for the attenuation properties of each ray sum and correlates them with the position of the ray. The result of this type of correlation is called an **attenuation profile.** An attenuation profile is created for each view in the scan. The information from all of the profiles is projected onto a

---

* Most scanners refer to this point as − 50, using numbers that are consecutively more negative as the scan progresses toward the feet. However, some systems reverse this numbering system. There are also systems that refer to this point as I50, meaning 50 mm inferior to the zero point.

A

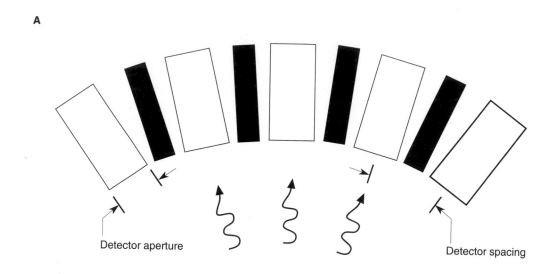

Detector aperture

Detector spacing

B

Scatter acceptance

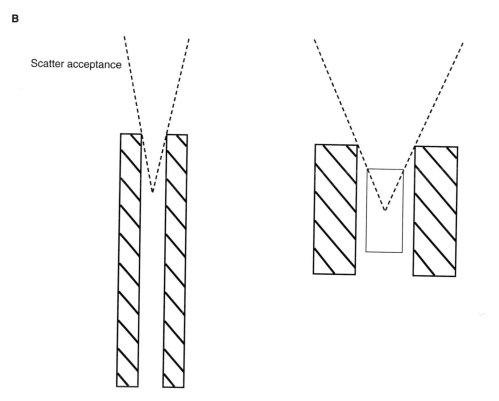

Fig. 2–5. Detector spacing and aperture. *(A)* The width and spacing of the detectors affect the amount of scatter that is recorded. *(B)* Low scatter acceptance is desirable. Simple geometric principles affect scatter acceptance.

matrix. This process of converting the data from the attenuation profile to a matrix is known as **back projection.**

There is a significant drawback to back projecting data onto a matrix: it produces streaks, or artifacts, on the image. To minimize these artifacts, a process called **filtering** is applied to the scanned data before back projection occurs. The process of filtering is done through complicated mathematic steps. The process of applying a filter function to an attenuation profile is called **convolution.** Different mathematic functions can be selected, depending on which parts of the data must be enhanced or suppressed. Depending on the manufacturer, the filter function may be referred to as algorithm, convolution filter, or CR filter.

Each time the x-ray tube is activated, information is gathered and fed into the system computer. The computer processes thousands of bits of data from each scan acquired to create the CT image. These data must be saved on a computer file so that the information will be available for use in the formation of an image. These stored data can later be retrieved and manipulated. The hard disk is the device within the computer that saves this information. The hard disk is an essential component of all CT systems. The number of images that the hard disk can store varies according to the make and model of the scanner. It is important to remember that an enormous amount of information is collected for each image.

For example, a single image in a 512 matrix system consists of 262,144 pixels (512 × 512). The digitization requires 10 to 12 bits; an 8-bit byte is standard. Therefore, it takes 2 bytes to cover each pixel in the dynamic range. This requirement translates to 2 × 262,144 = 524,288 bytes, or 0.52 megabytes (MB). When a 1024 matrix system is used, each image requires approximately 2 MB.

When the hard disk space capacity is reached, existing data must be deleted before any new data can be acquired. Many facilities use a long-term storage device to save these data. Saving studies on auxiliary devices for possible future viewing is referred to as **archiving.** The many options available for archiving are discussed in Chapter 8.

Raw Data

All of the thousands of bits of data acquired by the system with each scan are called **raw data.** The terms **scan data** and **raw data** are used interchangeably to refer to the data sitting in the computer and waiting to be made into an image. The process of using raw data to create an image is called **image reconstruction.** The reconstruction that is automatically produced during scanning is often called **prospective reconstruction.** The same raw data may be used later to generate a new image. This process is referred to as **retrospective reconstruction.**

Because raw data include all measurements obtained from the detector array, a variety of images can be created from the same data. Because raw data require a vast amount of hard disk space, CT systems offer limited disk space for storage of raw data.

Image Data

To form an image, the computer assigns one value (Hounsfield unit) to each pixel. This value, or density number, is the average of all measurements for that pixel. The two-dimensional pixel represents a three-dimensional portion of patient tissue. The pixel value represents the proportional amount of x-ray energy that passes through anatomy and strikes the detector. Once the data are averaged so that each pixel has one associated number, an image can be formed. The data included in this image are appropriately called **image data.** Image data require approximately one-fifth of the computer space needed for raw data. For this reason, CT systems may allow space for 3000 image data files, but only 355 raw data files.†

If only the image data are available, data manipulation is limited. Image data allow measurements such as Hounsfield units, standard deviation (see Chapter 5), and distance, but anything not seen on the image is unavailable for analysis.

Scan Field of View

Scan field of view is also called **calibration field of view.** Selecting the scan field of view determines the area, within the gantry, from which the raw data are acquired (see Figure 2–6). By selecting a 25-cm scan field of view, a technologist acquires data in a circular

---

† The proportion of image data to raw data files is specific to each make and model of scanner. The example used is for the Picker model PQ 2000SLR.

A

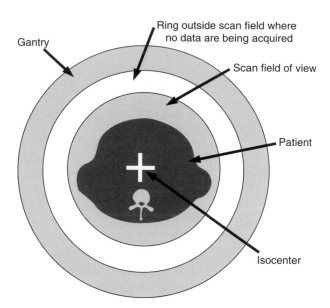

Gantry

Ring outside scan field where
no data are being acquired

Scan field of view

Patient

Isocenter

B

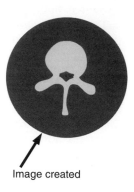

Image created

Fig. 2–6. *(A)* Raw data are collected within the scan field of view. *(B)* Image data are confined to those displayed on the monitor.

shape, with a diameter of 25 cm, lying in the absolute center, or **isocenter,** of the gantry. Because scan data are always acquired around the isocenter, the patient must be positioned in the center of the gantry. Scan field of view selection determines the number of detector cells collecting data. The choices of scan field of view vary among scanners. Typical choices are small (25 cm), which is used for the head; medium (35 cm), which is often used for the chest; and large (42–50 cm), which is used for the abdomen.

CT systems often incorporate other factors, in addition to size, into the scan field of view selection. These factors include calibration vectors and types of image processing (head versus body). It is important to understand which factors are being included with which scan field of view. For instance, if two small fields are available on a scanner, both offering a 25-cm scan size, how do they differ? Usually, the difference is related to associated image processing, which attempts to compensate for body part size (see Chapter 3). Choices specific to each manufacturer are described in the product literature.

Anything outside the scan field of view circle is not imaged because no data are collected beyond this circle.‡ To produce the highest quality image, the operator should select the scan field of view that comes closest to just encompassing the patient. It is important that no part of the patient lie outside the scan field. Parts of the patient located outside the scan field may cause inaccuracies in the image, called **out-of-field artifacts.** These artifacts cause streaking, shading, and incorrect Hounsfield numbers.

Data are not acquired on everything within the gantry. For example, if the gantry opening is 70 cm but the largest scan field of view available is 48 cm, there will be a ring where data cannot be collected.

Display Field of View

Selecting the **display field of view** (also called **zoom** or **target**) determines how

---

‡ A few systems collect data outside the field of view, but apply calibration only to the selected scan field size. In these systems, anatomy just outside the scan field of view will not cause significant artifacts.

much of the raw data are used to create an image. For example, if a lumbar spine is correctly scanned with a large scan field of view to include the entire body, but the operator chooses to target the image so that the vertebrae occupy most of the screen, the rest of the patient's abdomen is not visualized on the image. The section that is visualized is the display field of view. Increasing the display field of view increases the size of each pixel within the image. Because more information is packed into each pixel, a loss of resolution can result.

The display field of view and the matrix determine the pixel size. The size of the pixel can be determined by dividing the field of view by the matrix size.

$$\text{Pixel size} = \text{Field of view/Matrix size}$$

or

$$\text{Field of view} = \text{Pixel size} \times \text{Matrix size}$$

For example, if a viewer is looking at a grid through a camera lens and wishes to see the entire grid, she adjusts the lens of the camera to a corresponding point. If the viewer wishes to see a specific part of the grid more clearly, she adjusts the zoom of the camera lens to enlarge that part, even though other sections of the grid will no longer be visible. In the enlarged image seen through the camera lens, each square of the grid is larger, but no distortion of the grid occurs (see Figure 2–7). It is important to understand that changing the display field of view does not distort the resulting image. Postprocessing magnification of the image, which causes distortions, is discussed in Chapter 5. The example of the camera lens can be expressed as an equation as well. To summarize, targeted reconstruction (i.e., adjusting the field of view size) allows the operator to match the scanner resolution to pixel size. Magnification will only make the image larger.

Most scanners offer a variety of sizes for the display field of view. The operator selects one based on the examination being performed and the size of the patient.

CHAPTER SUMMARY

CT images are produced by x-ray beams that penetrate a patient and, to varying degrees, strike a detector. The placement of the x-ray tube relative to the detectors determines the generation of the scanner.

The CT process is broken down into three segments: data acquisition, image reconstruction, and image display.

To acquire data, a generator, gantry, and table are necessary. The generator supplies the energy source to the gantry. The x-ray tube, data acquisition system, collimators, and detectors are housed in the gantry.

Because of the number of exposures typical of a CT scanner and the high x-ray energy output of those scans, tubes must be designed

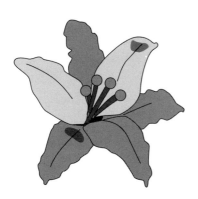
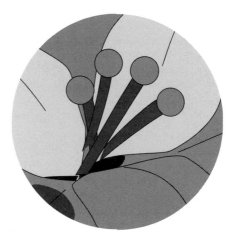

Fig. 2–7. Selecting the display field of view determines how much of the raw data are used to create an image. Display field works like the zoom on a camera and can be used to show the entire area or display a specific region of interest in greater detail.

to withstand huge amounts of heat. The amount of heat that the tube can withstand and the rate at which heat is dissipated are key factors in the cost of specific scanners.

Beam hardening artifacts occur because x-ray beams are not uniform in energy. These artifacts alter the image's Hounsfield values. Filters are included in most systems to reduce the amount of low-energy x-ray beams to reach the patient.

Source collimators operate like tiny shutters to allow only thin slivers of x-ray beams to emerge. The collimators can be adjusted by the operator. The low scatter radiation in CT scanning is attributed to this fine collimation.

Detectors are of two general types: pressurized xenon gas and solid-state crystals. When a solid-state crystal is struck by x-ray beams, it emits light. For this reason, these crystals are often referred to as scintillators. There are advantages and disadvantages to both types of detectors.

Raw data include all measurements obtained from the detector array. Some of these raw data are used in the creation of image data.

After the raw data are averaged and each pixel is assigned a Hounsfield number, an image can be reconstructed. The data that form this image are then referred to as image data.

Raw data occupy a great deal of disk space. For this reason, raw data space is limited.

Scan field of view refers to a selected circle in the center of the gantry. Raw data are acquired and calibrated for any object that lies within this circle. The entire scan circle or a portion of the circle may be selected to display on the monitor. The size of the circle that is displayed is called display field of view.

The pixel size is determined by dividing the field of view by the matrix size.

REVIEW QUESTIONS

1. What is milliampere level?
2. Define heat capacity and heat dissipation.
3. Why are solid-state detectors sometimes called scintillators?
4. What is the function of the data acquisition system?
5. What part of the CT system is often called the "brain" of the CT scanner?
6. How many Hounsfield units are assigned to each pixel in the image matrix?
7. What are the three segments of the CT process?
8. Explain the fundamental difference between third- and fourth-generation CT systems.
9. Define artifact.
10. What causes beam hardening artifacts?
11. How does filtration improve the CT image?
12. Define contrast resolution.
13. What is afterglow? Which type of detector does it affect?
14. Which type of detector is more efficient in its ability to capture transmitted photons and convert them to electric signals?
15. Why is it important for all CT staff to set landmarks in the same way?
16. What is back projection?
17. What is the difference between raw data and image data?
18. Why does the CT system's hard disk hold more image data files than raw data files?
19. Besides size, what might be included in a scan field of view selection?
20. How can out-of-field artifacts be avoided?

Chapter 3

FACTORS AFFECTING IMAGE QUALITY

SCANNING PARAMETERS

Many factors affect the quality of the image produced. Some of these variables can be regulated by the operator, whereas others, such as patient size, cannot.

Among the factors that the operator can control are milliampere (mA) level, scan time, slice thickness, field of view, and scan algorithm. On some systems, the operator may adjust the kilovolt-peak (kVp) setting, although on many systems, it is fixed at 120 kV. As a group, these factors are usually referred to as scanning parameters.

As in standard radiography, the total x-ray beam exposure in CT is dependent on a combination of milliampere setting, scan time, and kilovolt-peak setting. Milliampere level and scan time together define the quantity of x-ray energy, whereas **kilovolt-peak** setting defines the quality, or average energy, of the beam. These factors are analogous to water flowing through a hose. The intensity, or force, with which the water flows through the hose resembles kilovolt-peak level. The quantity of water that flows through the hose is similar to milliampere level. The length of time the water flows is similar to scan time. The product of milliampere setting and scan time is known as **milliampere-seconds** (mAs) and is the quantitative measure of the x-ray beam.

Milliampere-Second Setting

Within the x-ray tube are filaments, a cathode and an anode. These elements provide the electrons that create the x-ray beam. The system heats the filament until electrons start to "boil off" and break away from the filament. This current is measured in milliamperes. Increasing the number of milliamperes increases the number of electrons that make x-ray beams. Use of a small filament size concentrates the focal spot and improves spatial resolution. **Spatial resolution** is defined as the ability to present small objects and differ-

entiate between closely spaced objects. Unfortunately, small filaments cannot tolerate a high level of milliamperes. Therefore, systems that offer higher milliampere settings usually provide two separate filaments. A small filament is provided for lower milliampere settings (typically less than 200) and a large filament for higher settings. In reality, the loss of resolution caused by a larger filament is slight, and it is nearly impossible to see on a standard CT image.

Incorrect milliampere-second settings affect CT images differently than incorrect milliampere-settings in conventional radiography. This effect is caused by the large dynamic range of the detectors (up to 10,000:1) compared with film/screen radiography (approximately 100:1).

If too low a milliampere-second setting is used, the image does not appear too light, as would a chest x-ray. Rather, the underexposed CT image has a grainy appearance because an insufficient number of x-ray photons reach the detectors. An overexposed CT image is not seriously degraded, although some streaking artifacts are possible. The main concern in using more than the ideal milliampere-second setting is exposing the patient to unnecessary radiation.

An example illustrates the relation between milliampere setting and scan time. If 320 mAs is required for a specific study of the abdomen, this number can be obtained from a variety of combinations, based on the milliampere settings and scan times available with the specific system. For example, the selection of 80 mA and a 4-second scan time provides the same quantity of x-ray energy as 160 mA and a 2-second scan time.

Scanners vary in the milliampere settings that they offer. The previous example shows how higher milliampere settings allow shorter scan times to be used. This practice is critical in avoiding image degradation as a result of patient motion. Even with a cooperative patient who remains still and suspends respirations on command, motion can be a factor because of involuntary movement such as peristalsis and cardiac motion. Shorter scan times reduce, but do not eliminate, artifacts caused by motion. Therefore, if the total milliampere-second level can be maintained, it is generally preferable to use the shortest scan time available.

However, there are exceptions to this rule. Slower scan speeds are favored when monitoring the total expression of body movements for use in radiation therapy planning. In addition to this factor, many systems switch to a larger focal spot size as mA is increased. Theoretically, a larger focal spot could decrease spatial resolution. In reality, this effect is minimal.

As the milliampere-second level increases, so does the amount of heat being generated within the x-ray tube. This heat is a limiting factor in all scanners. On many systems, there is a direct correlation between milliampere-second level and interscan delay time. The higher the milliampere-second setting, the longer the time between scans while the tube cools off enough to allow another scan. On newer, top-of-the-line scanners, this delay is much less of a problem. In fact, maximum milliampere-second capabilities, minimum interscan delays, and corresponding heat dissipation rates are significant factors that distinguish scanners in various price ranges.

A number of factors affect which milliampere-second level is selected. These factors are basically the same as in conventional radiography. Specifically, the thicker and denser the part being examined, the more milliampere-seconds are required to produce an adequate image. For example, a CT study of the lungs will require less milliampere-seconds than that of the abdomen because the chest is composed primarily of the lungs, which contain air and are less dense than the organs of the abdomen.

Determining the optimal milliampere-second setting is often a matter of trial and error. Manufacturers often make general recommendations for the setting required for various examinations. There can be as great as a 20% difference in milliampere-second level before a visible change occurs on the image. For example, if the recommended setting for a specific study is 400 mAs, and the scanner has settings of 80, 100, and 130 mA as well as a choice of scan times of 3 or 5 seconds,

either 80 mA and 5 seconds (400 mAs) or 130 mA and 3 seconds (390 mAs) can be used. The 130-mA setting would probably be the first choice because of the decrease in motion related to the shorter scan time.

Scan Geometry

Another important factor is tube arc. Traditionally, a CT scan is considered one 360° rotation of the x-ray tube. In this case, two matching samples are taken 180° apart. These samples contribute similar information to the reconstructed image. By averaging the information from two similar views, the image is usually improved.

Although a 360° tube rotation per scan is the most common selection, it is not the only choice. It is possible to obtain a partial scan, which is acquired from 180° plus the degree of arc of the fan angle. Although this scan is slightly more than a half circle, these scans are often referred to as **half-scans.** Only half of the data are available to reconstruct the image with partial scans; therefore, they are inferior to standard 360° scans. However, these scans have a limited application in studies that require short scan times, such as pediatric studies.

Another tube arc option is the 400° scan, known as an **overscan.** The overscan adds approximately the width of the field of view to a full scan. These are more commonly used in fourth-generation scanner designs. In a stationary detector design, the views are not recorded instantaneously, but are taken over approximately one-fifth of the scan time. Because this timing increases the inconsistency of data within views, motion is more of a problem. This disadvantage can be minimized by using overscans. By allowing some overlap of data from the first and last tube positions, overscans reduce motion artifacts.

SLIP-RING SCANNERS

Slip-Ring Device

Recent developments in scanner design allow both the scan time and the time between scans (interscan delay) to be reduced. Among these developments, the one that has received the most attention is the **slip-ring** CT gantry. In this type of CT system, the gantry rotates continually in the same direction. In contrast, the conventional system makes a 360° rotation in one direction, comes to a complete stop, then turns 360° in the opposing direction. The slip-ring tube is also referred to as a **continuous rotation gantry.** Because the gantry does not require continuous stopping and starting, it can reach a much higher rotational speed within the gantry. Consequently, this higher rotational speed accounts for the reduced scan time. To maintain the same quality image, the milliampere setting must be increased when scan time is decreased.

To realize the greatest benefits from the slip-ring design, other hardware modifications became necessary. The development of quicker, smoother moving tables was essential in reducing the time between axial scans. Improving table features was vital in the development of continuous acquisition (also known as spiral, or helical) scanning (see Chapter 4). Improved tube cooling mechanisms and software that adjusts for motion were developed in conjunction with the slip-ring technology. New technologies are always reflected in the price. While there are a variety of slip-ring scanners on the market in a range of prices, slip-ring scanners are generally more expensive than conventional systems.

Kilovolt-Peak Setting

On many systems, the kilovolt-peak setting is fixed, typically at 120 kVp. Some systems have variable settings. Increasing the kilovolt-peak setting increases the intensity of the x-ray beam and the beam's ability to penetrate a thick, dense anatomic part. It may also decrease beam hardening artifacts because of the increase in the average photon energy. If higher kilovolt-peak settings are available, they are typically recommended for use in the posterior fossa and lumbar spine.

Slice Thickness

Slice thickness is important in CT. In general, thinner slices produce sharper images because, to create an image, the system must flatten the scan thickness (a volume) into two dimensions (a flat image). The thicker the slice, the more flattening is necessary. The system flattens the slice by taking the average of a cube (voxel) of tissue so that it can be represented as a square (pixel). The system produces an averaged, rather than absolutely accurate pixel value (Hounsfield unit). The greater the slice thickness, the more pronounced the inaccuracies, particularly in tissue that is heterogeneous. This effect is called **volume averaging** or **partial volume effect.**

Although the benefits of using thin slices in reducing volume averaging are considerable, there are significant drawbacks as well. One is that the radiation dose to the patient increases as slice thickness decreases. Thinner slices mean that more slices are needed to cover the same area, and the results are longer examination time, greater tube wear, use of more film, and higher associated costs.

Thin slices are used when the part being examined is small. For example, studies of the internal auditory canals are typically performed with the thinnest slice available (1–2 mm).

A narrower beam produces a smaller number of detected photons. Therefore, the milliampere-second level must increase as slice thickness decreases. If the milliampere-second level is not adjusted to compensate for the thinner slice, resulting images will have a grainy, or noisy, appearance.

Scanners vary somewhat in terms of available slice thicknesses. A slice between 1 and 2 mm thick is considered thin, whereas a thick slice is generally 8 to 10 mm. Intermediate thicknesses are also available.

Field of View

Selecting the correct scan field of view is important to reduce out-of-field artifacts (see Chapter 2). The improper selection of scan field of view can only be corrected by rescanning the patient.

Choosing the optimal display field improves the detectability of abnormalities. Selecting too large a display field makes the image appear unnecessarily small. In addition to the inherent difficulty in viewing smaller images, more information is provided in each pixel. For this reason, a small lesion may escape detection. On the other hand, too small a display field may exclude necessary patient anatomy.

Scanners are being designed to store more raw data. This capability permits the operator to correct an improper display field size by retrospectively reconstructing the data. It is important to view and evaluate images soon after their acquisition because raw data generally are not available for a long time.

Algorithm

Depending on the manufacturer, this feature may be called algorithm, convolution filter, CR filter, FC number, or simply filter. An algorithm is defined as any method of solving a certain type of problem. In CT, the problem is to recreate an image that accurately represents the object scanned. Current scanners offer several algorithm choices that are designed to reconstruct optimal images depending on tissue type.

By choosing a specific algorithm, the operator selects how the data are filtered in the reconstruction process. The process of filtering data is often called **convolution.** Each algorithm uses a different mathematic formula for processing data. This formula enhances certain features of the CT image. For example, if the operator selects a bone algorithm, the edges of anatomic structures are enhanced and a higher contrast image is provided. With the use of this filter, the resulting image may better visualize a bone deformity. This advantage is gained at the cost of reduced visability of the soft tissue structures, where the high-contrast filter produces a noisy effect. For this reason, certain studies require the data to be reconstructed with two separate algorithms. One optimizes low-contrast detectability in the soft tissue. The second provides optimal high spatial resolution and is preferable for bone. In general, high-contrast (also called bone, edge, detail, or sharp) algorithms are used to visualize structures with intrinsically high subject contrast, such as temporal bones or lung tissue. "Soft" algorithms are usually preferable for examining low-contrast areas, such as the brain and abdomen.

The best way to determine the optimal algorithm for any specific study is by experimentation. By using saved raw data, the same data can be retrospectively reconstructed into many images, each with a different algorithm. In a side-by-side comparison, it is much easier to determine which algorithm is best for a given application.

ARTIFACTS

Any object seen on the image that is not present in the object scanned is considered an artifact. A variety of sources cause artifacts. Recognizing the possible causes of artifacts can save a significant amount of time and money. Table 3-1 lists the most common artifacts, their typical causes, and steps that can be taken to resolve them. Ideally, better identification of artifacts can permit them to be corrected without a service call; or, if the severity of the artifact requires a service engineer, the call can be placed promptly.

CHAPTER SUMMARY

To a large extent, image quality can be controlled by the technologist. The factors that can be adjusted are milliampere setting, scan time, slice thickness, field of view, and algorithm. On some scanners, it is possible to adjust kilovolt-peak setting.

The amount of x-ray energy produced is known as milliampere level. The time span in which the beams are produced is the scan time. The product of these two factors is milliampere-seconds, which is the quantitative measure of x-ray beam exposure.

If insufficient milliampere-seconds are used, the result is a noisy, or grainy, image because too few x-ray photons strike the detectors.

The selection of specific milliampere and scan time settings is often a matter of compromise. It is important to evaluate the requirements of a specific examination before a decision is made. Small differences in milliampere-second level are usually not discernable on an image.

By producing more heat, higher milliampere-second settings place a greater burden on the x-ray tube.

The most commonly used scan makes a 360° arc within the gantry. However, scans that use a 180° arc (partial scans) and those that use a 400° arc (overscan) are also available.

The kilovolt-peak level is the measure of the energy of the x-ray beam. On most systems, this value is fixed at 120 kVp; however, some scanners offer a selection of settings. Increasing the kilovolt-peak setting increases the ability of the beam to penetrate a thick or dense anatomic part.

Slice thickness is primarily important for the part it plays in volume averaging. Thinner slices reduce volume averaging, but increase patient exposure. To avoid producing a noisy

Table 3–1.   Troubleshooting Artifacts on the CT Image

Manifestation	Possible Cause	Corrective Steps
Ring	Detector problem; more common on third-generation scanners because the tube and detector move together; rarely seen on fourth-generation systems	Recalibrate; if rings persist, call service
Aliasing effect (fine lines on image)	Too few samples	If partial scan was used, rescan with a complete arc; increase scan time
Edge gradient effect (straight line radiating from high-contrast areas, such as bone or soft tissue)	Angle of x-ray beam varies between two similar views	Increase scan time; decrease slice thickness
Beam hardening artifact [broad streaks, cupping (periphery of image is lighter), vague areas of low density]	X-ray beams are composed of different energies	Increase kilovolt-peak setting; decrease slice thickness; decrease milliampere level; increase filtration
Noise [grainy appearance (accentuated by narrow window levels)]	Insufficient photons reaching detectors; may be caused by low milliampere level, low tube output	Increase milliampere level; increase slice thickness; call service
Out-of-field artifacts (shading at the periphery of the image)	Patient is not entirely enclosed in scan field	Increase scan field size
Air–contrast interface artifact	Significant difference in density between contrast and air; motion may contribute; most frequent in gastric air–fluid level	Rescan patient in a decubitus or prone position if necessary
Lines on scout image	Faulty detector	Call service

image, it is necessary to increase milliampere-second level as slice thickness decreases.

Proper selection of scan field of view minimizes out-of-field artifacts. Display field of view affects lesion detectability. Display fields may be adjusted after a study is completed if the raw data are still available.

The mathematic process of filtering data is called an algorithm. Changing the algorithm may enhance certain image features. Correct algorithm selection is dependent on the type of study being performed.

Many types of artifacts exist in CT. More than one type of artifact may play a role in a specific image. All artifacts degrade the image. It is helpful to be able to identify the types and causes of artifacts. A service call is often necessary to correct artifacts caused by mechanical malfunctions.

REVIEW QUESTIONS

1. What factors are referred to as scanning parameters?

2. What factors define the quantity of x-ray energy produced?
3. What factor defines the intensity of the x-ray beam?
4. How does filament size affect image quality?
5. Define spatial resolution.
6. How is the CT image affected by too low a milliampere-second setting?
7. What is the major disadvantage of high milliampere settings?
8. Define partial scan and overscan.
9. How is a slip-ring scanner different from a traditional scanner?
10. What effect does slice thickness have on the radiation dose?
11. What other scanning parameter must be adjusted when slice thickness is decreased?
12. Why might a study be reconstructed in two different algorithms?
13. How can beam hardening artifacts be reduced?
14. What causes air–contrast interface artifacts?

Chapter 4

METHODS OF DATA ACQUISITION

New developments in CT scanning offer increased options for collecting data. These options are dependent on the model of scanner used. This chapter describes all scanning methods currently on the market: (1) standard axial scanning, (2) cluster scanning, (3) continuous acquisition scanning, and (4) cine scanning. More expensive scanners generally perform all methods, whereas lower-priced models typically are limited to conventional methods.

STANDARD AXIAL ACQUISITION TECHNIQUES

This method is the oldest and most widely used means of collecting data. It consists of: (1) having the patient suspend respiration (for body scans), (2) acquiring data for a single slice, (3) allowing the patient to resume normal breathing, (4) moving the table to the next slice location, and (5) repeating the procedure until the desired area is covered.

The characteristic that sets this system apart from other scanning methods is that the patient is allowed to breathe after each scan.

Historically, all scanners were designed to function this way. New scanners still function in a standard axial mode if desired. The time that is required to progress from step 1 to step 5 varies dramatically from scanner to scanner.

Scanners that function exclusively in this manner do so for a number of reasons. First, time is required for an x-ray tube to rotate in one direction, stop, then rotate in the opposite direction. Generally, a patient can only hold his breath for one revolution of the x-ray tube.

Second, a system may require the tube to cool before another scan can be obtained. This tube cooling takes 3 to 30 seconds. The patient must be allowed to breathe while the tube cools.

Third, some scanner systems do not permit sequential scans to be obtained while the computer reconstructs images and displays them. That is, these systems scan, reconstruct, then display. The entire cycle must be complete before the next image can be acquired. Such systems are referred to as **pipeline scanners.**

Slice Misregistration

A disadvantage of standard axial scanning is **slice misregistration,** which occurs when a patient breathes differently with each scan.

A shallow breath places the slice at a specific level of anatomy. The table is moved to the next scan position. The next scan is taken, but the patient takes a deep breath instead. This difference in breathing places the second scan in an incorrect anatomic position relative to the first slice. Valuable information may be missed because of this effect (see Figure 4-1).

To reduce the likelihood of slice misregistration, it is important to give the patient careful breathing instructions. The patient should be told that suspending respiration in an identical manner, every time he is asked, is crucial to completing a quality examination. However, even with precise instructions, significant slice misregistration may occur.

Dynamic Scanning

Dynamic scanning is a confusing term that is rapidly becoming obsolete. It has different meanings to different people. However, because it is often used, no CT text would be complete without an explanation of the different ways in which the term is used.

Early scanners often had interscan delay times of 30 seconds or more. Often, scanning within peak contrast enhancement was impossible because of these delays. Because of this disadvantage, dynamic scanning was born. In the truest sense of the word, dynamic scans refer to slices that are performed at a speed faster than the system's usual mode. This procedure is often accomplished by lowering the milliampere-second (mAs) level to

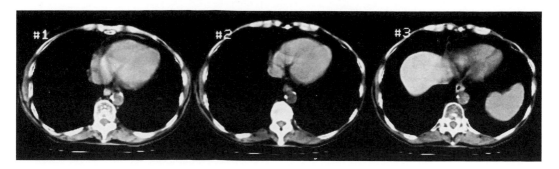

Fig. 4–1. Slice misregistration caused by patient breathing. Each consecutive slice was 10 mm more inferior, yet the second image appears the most superior. It is possible to miss lesions as large as 1 cm as a result of slice misregistration.

reduce tube cooling. On some scanners, it is possible to suspend image reconstructions and therefore speed scan acquisition. The liver is the most common organ selected for dynamic scanning. In this way, the liver can be scanned at peak contrast enhancement.

Dynamic scanning is often used in the diagnosis of liver hemangiomas. For this application, it is necessary to scan repeatedly at the same table position. This type of scanning is done to evaluate the enhancement of the suspected hemangioma. Liver hemangiomas typically appear as areas of low attenuation (darker), then after contrast enhancement, gradually become the same density (isodense) as normal liver tissue. Because of its common use in this manner, many practitioners incorrectly define dynamic scanning as rapid scanning done at the same level of anatomy.

Because new scanners are much faster, often performing routine scans faster than those once called dynamic, the term is becoming obsolete. In its place are the terms **rapid acquisition scanning** and **rapid scan.** If the scanning is done at the same level of anatomy, the descriptive term is **nonincremental scanning.**

CLUSTER SCANNING

Cluster scanning is the practice of grouping more than one scan in a single breath hold. Grouping scans in this way is possible because newer scanners are much faster than their predecessors. To illustrate this concept, the General Electric Hi-Speed scanner can produce an axial image every other second (1 second to acquire data; 1 second to move the table to the next position). It is not necessary to ask the patient to hold her breath to complete one scan because the system completes a group of scans in a single breath hold. The number of scans is dependent on how long the patient can hold her breath. For example, if a patient can suspend respiration for 11 seconds, a cluster of six scans may be performed before the patient is instructed to breathe (6 seconds for data acquisition; 1 second between each scan for table movement). The number of scans per cluster and the breathing time between clusters are programmable features that are dependent on each patient's condition.

The primary advantage of this method of scanning is the reduction in slice misregistration. Another benefit is decreased examination time. Patients generally prefer this method because they are not required to hold their breath as frequently.

A disadvantage of scanning at increased speeds is that image reconstruction cannot keep up with data acquisition. Therefore, the image displayed on the monitor can lag significantly behind the slice that is being taken. The routine of watching images as they appear and making adjustments accordingly is not practical when scanning at this increased rate.

The industry as a whole is attempting to increase the speed of image reconstruction. This disadvantage may be overcome as the technology progresses.

Pancreas scanning provides a good example of how rapid scanning may change the existing protocol. Traditionally, the diaphragm is scanned with a 10-mm slice thickness. The technologist watches the images as

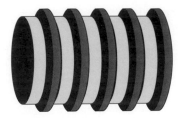

Fig. 4–2. Axial slices lie parallel to one another. The slice beginning matches exactly the slice end, and perfect rings are formed.

they appear on the monitor, and when the first sign of the pancreas is detected, the scanner is paused and the slice thickness is adjusted to 5 mm. With fast scanning methods, this practice is no longer realistic. By the time the first slice of the pancreas is displayed on the screen, the entire examination is completed.

To accommodate the faster scan speed, it is necessary to adjust the scanning routine. For the pancreas, the location is estimated from the scout image, and the thinner slices are prescribed before the examination begins. The disadvantage of this change is that because the location is only estimated, more slices than absolutely necessary may be taken. Whether this type of trade-off is justifiable depends on the workload and philosophy of each facility.

CONTINUOUS ACQUISITION SCANNING

Usually known as **spiral,** or **helical,** scanning, continuous acquisition scanning is the

most important CT innovation in years. Scanners that offer the option of spiral scanning are also capable of producing scans with the traditional axial method. The spiral method uses a continually rotating x-ray gantry with constant x-ray output and uninterrupted table movement. In certain instances, 60 images can be acquired in 1 minute.

Because the data are acquired continually as opposed to the start-and-stop method used in conventional axial scanning, the result is a volume, or block, of data. Acquiring a volume of information allows images to be manipulated in ways not available with conventional acquisition methods. Although the result is a block of data, it is important to remember that this information is acquired in thin ribbons, not one block at a time. Inherent limitations in data manipulation are discussed later in this chapter.

Numerous advancements make this technology possible: (1) x-ray gantries with a slip-ring design, (2) more efficient tube cooling, (3) higher x-ray output (increased milliampere capability), (4) smoother table movement, (5) software that adjusts for table motion, (6) improved raw data management, and (7) more efficient detectors.

Although virtually indistinguishable in appearance, the images produced by this method are not precisely axial. An axial image is taken so that each slice is parallel to every other slice, like bracelets on a wrist (see Figure 4–2). With a spiral technique, the images are similar to a spring, with each slice at a slight angle (see Figure 4–3).

The earliest spiral scanners required 1 second for the gantry to make a complete 360°

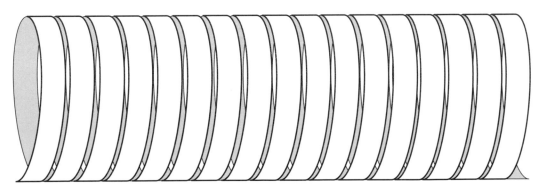

Fig. 4–3. Spiral scans are not precisely axial because their beginning slices do not match their end slices. Therefore, the slices are at a slight angle.

rotation. This feature was not adjustable. If the scan time is fixed, a higher range of milliampere settings is essential to maintain an appropriate milliampere-second level. In general, to offer a higher range of milliampere settings, it is necessary to increase both the size of the generator and the tube cooling capabilities of the system. These modifications significantly increase the cost of the CT system.

To keep the cost of a spiral system within the moderate price range, some companies offer spiral systems that compensate for lower milliampere setting options by slowing the tube rotation. Slowing the tube rotation from 1 to 2 seconds doubles the milliampere-second level. Obviously, examination time and motion artifact increase as scan time increases.

Scanning Formula

Regardless of the time required for the x-ray tube to make a complete rotation, in most cases, each image requires data from one complete rotation of the tube, as expressed by the formula:

$$\text{Total acquisition time} \times \frac{1}{\text{Rotation time}}$$
$$= \text{Number of images}$$

and

$$\text{Total acquisition time} \times \frac{1}{\text{Rotation time}}$$
$$\times \text{Slice thickness}$$
$$= \text{Amount of anatomy covered}$$

This formula assumes that the pitch is 1:1. Pitch is discussed later in this chapter.

According to this formula, a scan that is programmed for 30 seconds (total spiral acquisition time) with a technique that requires 1 second for each rotation of the x-ray tube (rotation time) produces 30 images. If this procedure uses a 10-mm slice thickness, 300 mm of anatomy is covered. That is:

30-second acquisition time

$$\times \frac{1}{\text{1-second rotation time}}$$
$$\times \text{10-mm slice thickness}$$
$$= 300 \text{ mm anatomy covered}$$

Changing Slice Incrementation Retrospectively

An advantage of spiral scanning is the ability to change the reconstructed slice incrementation. Because the data are acquired continually, raw data can be reconstructed retrospectively at any point. In this way, staggered slices can be created with as little as 1 mm difference.

In Figure 4–4A, the line represents a 5-second spiral scan performed with a 10-mm slice thickness. The system begins scanning at table position 0. An image is created from each second of tube travel; each image corresponds to 10 mm of patient anatomy. Therefore, image 1 is created from data that correlate to the anatomy at table positions 0 to 10. Image 2 is created from data that correlate to the anatomy at positions 10 to 20, and so on. Assume a low-density area is visualized on images 2 and 3, and the partial volume effect is suspected of creating an inaccurate Hounsfield measurement (see Chapter 1 for an explanation of partial volume effect). In an effort to reduce this effect, the raw data can be used retrospectively to create another image (see Figure 4-4B). This new image 6 correlates to the anatomy at table positions 15 to 25 (half of image 2 and half of image 3). The goal of this approach is to show the abnormality on only one image. Because this method reduces the normal tissue that is averaged in, the measurement is more accurate.

These reconstructions can be staggered by as little as 1 mm; in this way, an additional 90 images can be created from the same 10 seconds of data. Creating a series of overlapping images produces superior three-dimensional and multiplanar reformatted images and can be done without increased radiation exposure to the patient (see Chapter 5).

Although the slice incrementation can be changed with the raw data, it is impossible to change the actual slice thickness because the data are obtained in ribbons, and not a block at a time. As explained in Chapter 2, slice thickness is controlled by the physical opening of the collimator and cannot be changed retrospectively. The only way to obtain a thinner slice is to rescan the area.

Effective Slice Thickness

In contrast to traditional axial scanning, spiral scans gradually index down as the series progresses. Because the slice beginning does

A

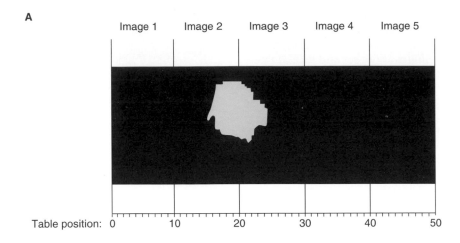

B

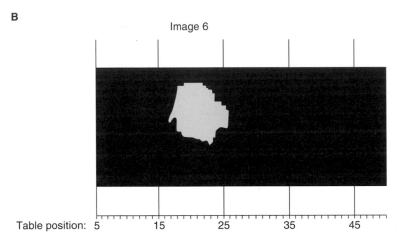

Fig. 4–4. Retrospectively changing the incrementation of spiral data can reduce the partial volume effect.

not match the slice end, each rotation is at a slight angle (see Figure 4–5). Computer software adjusts for this slight angle by averaging the data and creating an image that is not slanted. This software process is referred to as **interpolation** and is a complex statistical method of processing data. Different interpolation formulas are used and have varying degrees of accuracy. Interpolation allows for an accurate approximation of data that have not been acquired. It is similar to an educated guess.

Because of this software interpolation, the effective slice thickness is greater than the collimator opening. The degree to which the slice thickness is enlarged is dependent on

the efficiency of the software. The effect is negligible when a pitch of 1:1 is used (pitch is discussed later in this chapter). To summarize, slice thickness is affected to varying degrees and is dependent on pitch selection, selected slice thickness, and manufacturer. However, no system eliminates this problem inherent in continuous acquisition scanning.

Another problem occurs because the system must interpolate data to produce a spiral scan image. Any interpolation causes a slight decrease in image resolution and a resulting loss in detail. In reality, this effect is minimal and is more than offset by the benefits of scanning at peak contrast enhancement. In most cases, an axial image and a spiral image appear

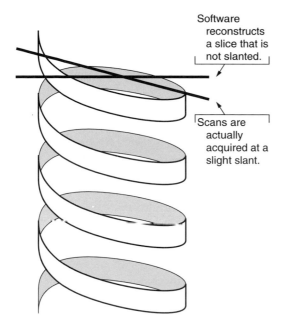

Software reconstructs a slice that is not slanted.

Scans are actually acquired at a slight slant.

Fig. 4–5. Spiral scans are acquired at a slight slant because of the continuous motion of the x-ray tube and table. The computer then creates an image that is not slanted by interpolating the data. This process increases the effective slice thickness and causes some loss of image resolution. The more pronounced the slant, the more interpolation is required. The slant is affected by selected slice thickness and pitch.

identical. Effective slice thickness and image noise are influenced by table pitch.

Pitch

The relation of table speed to slice thickness is referred to as **pitch.** With a pitch of 1:1, the table moves at a speed that allows all anatomic areas to be covered. That is, if the slice thickness is set at 5 mm, the table moves at a speed that allows the *gantry* to rotate once every 5 mm of table travel. If the pitch is adjusted to 2:1 and the slice thickness is maintained at 5 mm, the tube rotates only once for every 10 mm of table motion. This procedure is similar to stretching a spring (see Figure 4-6).

It would seem that using any pitch greater than 1:1 would result in data being skipped. This assumption is only partially true. The computer system is equipped with a feature that interpolates data for the missed information, so a scan is still produced for each table position. This practice is the equivalent of guessing at missed information based on the information that is acquired above and below the absent data. Because increasing the pitch increases the slant of each rung of the spiral, fewer data are collected for each table position.

Pitch is most often set at 1:1 so that data are not missed. Increasing pitch increases the effective slice thickness because more information must be interpolated to produce an image. Increasing effective slice thickness decreases image resolution. Pitch is directly proportional to effective slice thickness as well as resolution.

There are several reasons why pitch may be adjusted. Increasing pitch is sometimes used to speed scanning for pediatric patients or patients with acute trauma. Pitch may also be increased when covering a longer anatomic area in the shortest time possible is of paramount importance, such as the case in CT angiography. Another rationale for increasing pitch is to cover more data in each patient breath hold, thereby reducing slice misregistration. Increasing the pitch will reduce total

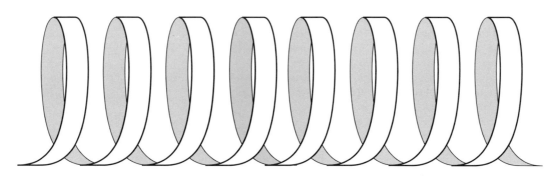

Fig. 4–6. The effect of increasing the pitch in a spiral scan.

radiation dose to the patient. On some scanners, it is possible to decrease pitch to less than 1:1. In such cases, the table moves more slowly so that the data are actually overlapping, with some areas of anatomy being exposed twice. This technique is sometimes employed to compensate for the increase in effective slice thickness. Although this approach improves image resolution, it involves greater radiation exposure to the patient.

The earlier equation can be modified to include a change in pitch. To account for a change in pitch, the entire equation is multiplied by the pitch.

$$\text{P} \times \text{Total acquisition time}$$
$$\times \frac{1}{\text{Rotation time}}$$
$$\times \text{Slice thickness}$$
$$= \text{Amount of anatomy covered}$$

Using the previous example, but changing the pitch to 2:1, the equation is:

$$\frac{2}{1} \times 30 \text{ second} \times \frac{1}{1 \text{ second}} \times 10 \text{ mm}$$
$$= 600 \text{ mm}$$

Pitch is expressed as a ratio of the velocity of the table to the rotational velocity of the x-ray tube.

or

$$\frac{\text{Velocity of table}}{\text{Rotational velocity of x-ray tube}}$$

Because the units of velocity cancel themselves out in the ratio, pitch need not be expressed in any unit.

It is important to weigh the inherent advantages and disadvantages whenever pitch is altered from 1:1. As the pitch increases from 1:1 toward 1.5:1, there is an associated loss of image resolution. As the pitch increases past 1.5:1 up to 2:1, the loss of resolution is much more dramatic.

Milliampere-Second Limitations

To maintain image quality, spiral scanning requires at least as high a milliampere-second level as traditional axial images. Because the scan time options are limited, it is sometimes difficult to maintain an appropriate milliampere-second level. If this level is not maintained, quantum noise results, as in axial images.

Manufacturers address this problem to some degree by improving the efficiency of the detectors. Improved detector efficiency allows a reduction in overall milliampere-second level on both axial and spiral scans.

Manufacturers also compensate for this problem by increasing the milliampere setting selection available. This modification requires a larger generator and increases the overall cost of the system.

Because of the limitation imposed by shorter scan times, spiral scanning is generally confined to small and medium patients. On large patients, the clinician has to decide if the added speed and contrast attained from spiral scanning outweigh the increase in noise.

Tube Cooling Limitations

Heat dissipation is a problem with all types of x-ray systems, from a portable x-ray unit to an angiographic suite. In spiral scanning, it is a major concern. Continuous x-ray production generates a tremendous amount of heat. Even a short time for tube cooling (such as the 1-second interscan delay in fast axial scanning) has a great effect on heat dissipation. The principles of standard x-ray physics apply to spiral scanning. That is, heat generated is directly proportional to milliampere-second level. In spiral scanning, the scan time is as high as 60 seconds. However, to scan for such long periods and consequently cover more anatomy per scan, the milliampere setting must be lowered. The technologist must maintain the setting above the minimum exposure necessary to produce a satisfactory image. Speed rarely takes precedence over image quality.

Like cluster scanning, some systems allow the technologist to break spiral scans into groups to allow the patient to breathe. This practice also allows some time for the tube to cool so that higher milliampere settings can be used.

An example of such a protocol is three groups of 12-second spiral scans, with 7-second intervals to allow for breathing. The total data acquisition time is 50 seconds; that is

$(12 \times 3) + (7 \times 2) = 50$. This time does not include image reconstruction time, only actual scanning time.

Effect on Total Scan Time and Contrast Dosage

When comparing spiral scanning with traditional axial scans (scan times of 2–5 seconds), spiral scanning reduces total examination time by more than 50%. To make such comparisons, it is necessary to factor in the time needed to repeat the command, "hold your breath."

Slower scanning procedures require more contrast medium to ensure that contrast enhancement is adequate throughout the examination. Some studies suggest that iodine dosage may be reduced by as much as 40% with spiral scanning. However, when fast axial slices (1- or 2-second scan time, with interscan delays of less than 3 seconds) are compared with spiral scanning, there is no appreciable difference in contrast dose.

Scanning at higher speeds requires contrast injection techniques to be exact. A difference of 30 seconds can mean that little contrast enhancement is visualized on the images, most commonly when scanning is begun too soon after injection. The first scan shows contrast, but it is absent on all subsequent images because the system can scan faster than the contrast can travel through the body (see Chapter 7).

Effect on Slice Misregistration and Motion

Slice misregistration is reduced because the patient is not required to hold his breath as often. There is also a reduction in motion caused by peristalsis and cardiac movement. This decrease occurs because each image is created from just 1 second of scanning. An overall reduction in gross patient motion is usually realized because patients can better tolerate a shorter examination.

Basic Spiral Scan Procedure

Spiral scanning is accomplished in the same way as axial slices: (1) a scout image is obtained; (2) the location of the spiral images are determined from the scout image; (3) the patient is asked to hold her breath (for body studies); (4) data are acquired in varying amounts, depending on the type of scan; (5) the patient is allowed to breathe; (6) steps 3 through 5 are repeated until all areas of interest are covered; and (7) the data are reconstructed into images that are displayed on the monitor.

Advantages and Disadvantages

The advantages of spiral scanning are: (1) increased speed, (2) a resultant need for less contrast material, (3) less slice misregistration, (4) reduced motion, (5) ability to change slice incrementation retrospectively, and (6) improved three-dimensional and multiplanar reformations.

The disadvantages inherent in spiral scanning are: (1) slightly thicker slice than selected (when pitch is greater than 1:1); (2) increased image noise if the milliampere setting cannot be maintained because of tube limit; (3) loss of image resolution because of the interpolation required to process spiral data; and (4) need for precise timing of contrast material injection.

CINE IMAGING

Cine imaging is defined as continuous acquisition scanning without table movement. The clinical applications for this feature are limited. They consist predominantly of observing arterial contrast enhancement in the heart and large vessels. Some systems allow each second of data to be retrospectively reconstructed into ten images, each representing one-tenth of a second. In the future, there may be a wider use for this feature in the evaluation of heart disease.

CHAPTER SUMMARY

Scanning options vary depending on the manufacturer. The most widely used option is standard axial scanning, which requires the patient to hold her breath for each scan. Slice misregistration is a disadvantage of this method.

The term dynamic scanning is becoming obsolete as a result of technologic improvements. Faster scanners can perform cluster scans in which the patient holds his breath for a group of axial scans. This technique reduces both total examination time and slice misregistration.

Continuous acquisition scanning is more commonly called helical or spiral scanning. It consists of a continuously rotating x-ray tube and uninterrupted table movement. Scanners must have a slip-ring design to scan in this way. Images appear identical to axial images, but possess some fundamental differences. There are definite trade-offs when comparing spiral scans with fast axial scans. Data incrementation can be changed on spiral scan data, but actual slice thickness cannot be adjusted retrospectively.

Pitch is the relation of table speed to slice thickness. Adjusting the pitch stretches or compresses the spiral. Pitch affects both effective slice thickness and image resolution.

Often, spiral scanning is limited to small and medium patients because of limitations in milliampere-second level. Total scan time is dramatically reduced with spiral scanning protocols. Because the total examination time is reduced, it is often possible to decrease the contrast material dosage by as much as 40%. In addition, scanning may be timed to coincide with peak contrast enhancement. Slice misregistration and motion artifact decrease with spiral techniques. Disadvantages include increased effective slice thickness because of the interpolation that is required to process spiral data. This interpolation also results in loss of image resolution.

REVIEW QUESTIONS

1. What causes slice misregistration?
2. What is the major advantage in clustering scans?
3. What advances make continuous acquisition scanning possible?
4. A spiral study is programmed with 2:1 pitch, 5-mm slice thickness, and 30-second total acquisition time. Each rotation of the tube requires 1 second. How much anatomy will be covered?
5. When is changing slice incrementation in a spiral study advantageous?
6. In a spiral study, why is it impossible to change slice thickness retrospectively?
7. What is interpolation?
8. Define pitch as it is used in spiral scanning.
9. How does an increase in pitch affect image resolution and effective slice thickness?
10. Why is it more difficult to maintain a sufficient milliampere-second level in spiral scanning as opposed to traditional axial scanning?
11. How does heat dissipation affect the spiral scanning process?
12. What are the advantages and disadvantages of spiral scanning compared with traditional axial scanning?

Chapter 5

IMAGE DISPLAY

WINDOW SETTINGS

The way an image is viewed on the computer monitor can be adjusted by changing the window width and window levels. At certain window settings, a slice of the thorax shows the lung parenchyma. At another setting, the same slice shows mediastinal detail and no longer displays the lung parenchyma. Many studies, such as those of the thorax, require each image to be scanned at two or more different window settings.

This chapter provides a technical explanation of window width and window levels. Although there are some guidelines for window settings, a substantial factor is personal preference. Ideally, windows should be set so that the radiologist responsible for interpretation is satisfied. In practice, it is often impossible for a technologist to know which physician will be responsible for interpreting any given examination. Therefore, it is best to establish general guidelines for the entire group of radiologists. It is well worth the radiologists' time to work closely with technologists to ensure that all parties understand exactly how the image is best displayed. It is essential that the technologists be allowed some discretion in setting windows. Factors such as patient size and body composition have a pronounced effect on window settings. Optimal images cannot be achieved with standardized window widths and levels that do not consider controlling factors. To produce consistently high-quality images, settings must be adjusted according to the specific circumstances.

Gray Scale

CT images are displayed on a cathode-ray tube (CRT) monitor. This monitor is basically a standard television set with some modifications that improve image resolution. Although there are more than 4000 different Hounsfield values, the monitor can display only 256 shades of gray. The human eye can differentiate only approximately 20 shades of gray. To overcome these inherent limitations, a gray scale is used in image display. This system assigns a certain number of Hounsfield units (HU) to each level of gray. The number of Hounsfield units assigned to each level of gray is determined by the window width.

As was explained in Chapter 1, the Hounsfield scale represents the density of water as 0. Correspondingly, -1000 HU represents air and 1000 HU represents a dense material, such as bone or contrast medium. Values from 2000 to 4000 HU represent very dense materials, such as steel. The gray scale assigns higher Hounsfield values lighter shades of gray, whereas lower numbers are represented by darker shades.

Window Width

The **window width** determines the range of Hounsfield units represented on a specific image (see Figure 5-1). The software assigns shades of gray to CT numbers that fall within the range selected. All values higher than the selected range appear white, and any value lower than the range appears black. By increasing the window width, usually referred to as "widening the width," more numbers are assigned to each shade of gray.

In general, wide window levels (400-2000 HU) are best for imaging tissue types that vary greatly when the goal is to see all of the various tissues on one image. For example, in lung imaging, it is necessary to see low-density lung parenchyma as well as high-density vascular structures. Wider windows encompass greater anatomic diversity, but subtle density discrimination is lost.

Tissue types with similar density should be displayed in a lower, or narrow, window width (50-400 HU). This approach is best in the brain, in which there is not as much variation in CT numbers. Because narrow widths provide greater density discrimination and

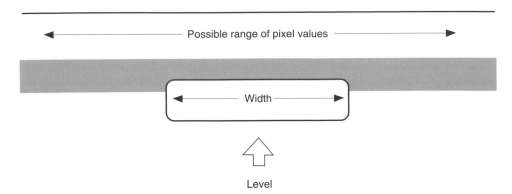

Fig. 5–1. Window width assigns the quantity of pixel values to the gray scale. Window level determines the center pixel value in the gray scale.

contrast, it is possible to differentiate the white and gray matter of the brain.

Because wider window settings decrease contrast, they suppress the display of noise on an image. For this reason, it is common practice to widen the window when patients are obese or when there are metallic artifacts.

Window Level

The **window level** selects the center CT value of the window width (see Figure 5-1). The terms window level and **window center** are often used interchangeably. The window level selects which Hounsfield numbers are displayed on the image.

For example, if a window width on a particular image is set at 300, which 300 of the more than 4000 possible Hounsfield numbers are represented? The answer is entirely dependent on which window level is selected. If 0 is chosen as the window level, the Hounsfield values range from − 150 to 150 on this image. Any value lower than − 150 appears black, whereas any value higher than 150 appears white. If the level is increased to 200, the range of visualized Hounsfield values is modified to between 50 and 350.

The window level should be set at a point that is roughly the same value as the average attenuation number of the tissue of interest. Each scanning protocol has a suggested window width and level for filming. This suggested setting is only approximate because preference varies enormously. Also, settings vary greatly according to patient size and body composition.

Some systems provide the option of recording two different window settings, superimposed on one another, in a single image. This technique is known as **dual window setting,** or **double window setting.** Dual window setting reduces the amount of film used compared with recording the window settings separately. However, because many professionals find this superimposition confusing and distracting, this technique is not often used in routine recording procedures.

IMAGE MAGNIFICATION

It is important to differentiate between image magnification and decreasing field of view size. A decrease in display field of view increases image size. The result of both functions is an image that appears larger than the original. In each case, relevant clinical data may be easier to see because of the enlargement. However, image magnification uses only image data, not raw data, and has the effect of stretching the image to a larger size. Magnification does not improve resolution, and image distortion rises with an increase in the magnification factor. In spite of these drawbacks, in many instances, simply magnifying the image data is appropriate. An example is the display of suspected abnormalities for measurement. Image magnification does not adversely affect the accuracy of Hounsfield unit or distance measurement. In fact, because magnifying the image may clarify the margins of the abnormality, allowing for more accurate cursor placement, measurement accuracy may improve.

Image magnification should not be used when the image displayed on the monitor appears too small. This problem results from inappropriate field size selection, and it should be corrected by using the raw data to reconstruct the entire study in the correct field size. Image resolution is improved if the image is enlarged using the raw data. However, if the raw data are not available, a less attractive alternative is to magnify each image in the study.

In summary, magnification is a useful tool that should be employed on isolated images within a study. Magnification allows relevant clinical detail to be more easily seen and more accurately measured. However, magnification has inherent limitations and should not be used as an alternative to correct display field selection.

Region of Interest

A display function available on all scanners is that of defining an area on the image. This area is referred to as the region of interest (ROI). An ROI is most often circular, but may be elliptic, square, or rectangular, or may be custom drawn by the operator. Defining the size, shape, and location of the ROI is the first step in many display and measurement functions. Image magnification, obtaining an averaged Hounsfield measurement, and acquiring the standard deviation all demand defining an ROI.

HOUNSFIELD MEASUREMENTS AND STANDARD DEVIATION

For the reasons mentioned previously, caution must be used when applying Hounsfield values in the diagnosis of pathology. However, Hounsfield measurement is one of several valuable tools that aid in diagnosis.

On most systems, a cursor ($+$) placed over an area reads out a measurement of that area. If a cursor is used, it is essential to understand that the subsequent measurement is only for the pixel covered by the cursor. If an ROI is first placed over an area, the reading is the average for all of the pixels within the ROI. If the ROI is accurately placed within the area of the suspected lesion, the averaged value is probably more accurate than the single-pixel reading.

A cursor measurement is effective when used as a rapid method of evaluating the density of a specific structure on an image. For example, if a cursor is placed over a known vascular area, such as the aorta, on the first image taken after the initiation of contrast media, this measure indicates whether the anatomy is actually contrast enhanced. If the measurement is 70 HU (indicating unenhanced blood) instead of the expected higher value of contrast-enhanced blood (90–120 HU), then a number of steps could be taken before the examination is continued. These steps may include checking the injection site for intravenous infiltration or checking the tubing for kinks, and increasing the delay between injection and the start of scanning because the contrast material has not reached the desired areas of the anatomy. Injection techniques are discussed in Chapter 7.

ROI measurements should be used whenever the values will be considered in formulating a diagnosis. When an area is used, in addition to the averaged Hounsfield value of the pixels within the ROI, a standard deviation reading is given. This reading indicates the amount of CT number variance within the ROI. For example, if an area of interest has a Hounsfield value of 5 and the standard deviation is 0, what is known about the region? This standard deviation shows that there is no variation within the ROI; therefore, every pixel within the region has the value of 5 HU. If the standard deviation is not 0, but 20, all of the pixels within the ROI do not have an identical reading of 5 HU. The higher the standard deviation, the greater the variation between pixels within the region.* The standard deviation does not indicate the levels of the individual pixels. Factors that produce high standard deviations are: (1) mixed attenuation tissue within the ROI (e.g., calcium flecks within an organ); (2) an ROI that includes a

---

* The standard deviation is the most widely used statistical measure of the spread or dispersion of a set of data. It is the positive square root of the variance. The standard deviation, like the variance, measures dispersion about the mean as center. However, the standard deviation has the same unit of measurement as the observation, whereas the unit of variance is the square of the unit of the observation. The standard deviation is always greater than or equal to zero. It is zero when all observations have the same value; this value is thus the mean, and so the dispersion is zero. The standard deviation increases as the dispersion increases. Mosteller FR, et al: *Probability with Statistical Applications*, 2nd ed. 1970.

streak artifact; and (3) an ROI that is not inside the margins of the object being measured (e.g., kidney cyst measured with an inappropriately large ROI that includes a section of the adjacent renal calyx, which is averaged in with the cyst). In the last two instances, the high standard deviation also reflects a less accurate Hounsfield measurement.

DISTANCE MEASUREMENTS

All CT systems allow distance measurements. This feature is helpful in reporting the size of the abnormality. It is also essential for the placement of a biopsy needle or drainage apparatus. The system calculates the distance between two deposited points in either centimeters or millimeters. Additionally, CT systems calculate the degree of angulation of the measurement line from the horizontal or vertical plane. A grid can also be placed over an entire image.

All CT images have a scale placed alongside the image for size reference. This feature allows a ruler to be placed along the scale, then subsequently placed along an area of pathologic tissue. The CT distance scale is used in the same way as a scale of miles in a map key.

PRIORITY RECONSTRUCTION

In new top-of-the-line scanners, acquisition speed is substantially faster than image reconstruction speed. In these cases, a backlog of raw data are waiting to be made into images. A convenient option available on many systems is selecting which data will be reconstructed first. With this function, a technologist can check the first few images of a study, then skip to the last image to determine whether the study ends at the anticipated location. Prioritizing reconstructions in this manner may increase department throughput. This feature may be called priority reconstruction, instant image, or urgent image, depending on the manufacturer.

IMAGE ANNOTATION

Typical information that appears on each image includes facility name, patient name, identification number, date, slice number and thickness, table location, measurement scale, gray scale, and right and left indicators. Often, other information is displayed as well. Optional information includes the addition of contrast enhancement and all scan parameter selections.

Software also allows the operator to annotate specific images with words, phrases, arrows, or other markers. Whenever computer software is used to alter the position of an image, an explanatory annotation is recommended. An example is recording a sinus study. If sinus studies are typically obtained in a coronal position, with the patient lying prone, and a specific study must be done with the patient reversed in the supine coronal position, images are often reversed for filming. It is important to note this change to prevent any potential misdiagnoses because fluid appears to be floating to the top.

REFERENCE IMAGE

The reference image function displays the slice lines in corresponding locations on the scout image. This feature aids in localizing slices according to anatomic landmarks.

MULTIPLE IMAGE DISPLAY

The multiple image display function allows more than one image to be displayed in a single frame. It is often used as a method of saving film, particularly when copies are requested by the referring physician. The formats (i.e., four images per frame, six images per frame) often vary with the manufacturer.

ADVANCED DISPLAY FUNCTIONS

Display and measurement functions that have more specialized applications are generally referred to as **advanced display functions.** On older scanners, most of these functions were cumbersome and time consuming and therefore were not frequently used. However, most newer scanners can perform these functions in a matter of seconds, so their use is becoming more common.

Histogram

A histogram displays a bar graph to show how frequently a range of CT numbers occurs within an ROI (see Figure 5–2).

Pixel Value

The pixel value function displays and identifies the CT numbers for a certain area. The

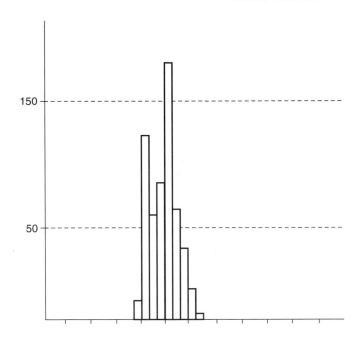

Fig. 5–2. The appearance and frequency of a range of CT numbers within a region of interest are displayed on a histogram.

area varies with the type of software. The center of the area is where the operator places the cursor.

Correlate

The correlate function allows areas on consecutive images to be traced, with their outlines then superimposed over the scout image (see Figure 5–3). Relating a specific area of abnormality to a known landmark is advantageous in surgical or radiation treatment planning.

Reformation

The process of using image data to create a view in a different body plane is called **reformatting.** Once again, the slice of bread analogy is helpful for clarification of the process. If the slices of bread are stacked so that they resemble an intact loaf and the loaf is cut in a different fashion (e.g., diagonally), the slices of bread can be seen from a new perspective. This example shows that all of the original slices of bread must have some common features to facilitate stacking them into a loaf. For example, they must be the same size, their edges must all match up, they must have the same original slice angle, and there must be no missing slices. Similarly, to successfully reformat a CT study, all slices must

have an identical display field of view, image center (i.e., the x, y coordinates must be the same), and gantry tilt, and they must be contiguous (i.e., no nonimaged spaces between slices). Because lining up the images exactly is vital in reformation, even a small amount of motion seriously degrades the end product.

Multiplanar Reformation

Reformation that is done to show the body in various body planes is referred to as **multiplanar reformation.** Many systems offer a feature known as **real-time reformation** that allows the operator to change the body plane while the software continually updates the image. This feature permits the operator to use trial and error to obtain the ideal image plane. Another common feature included in reformation software is the ability to create additional reformatted images from the first reformat. This reformatting from a reformat is helpful in imaging the lumbar spine. If the original images are taken with no gantry tilt through the disk space, a sagittal reformatted image is obtained (see Chapter 8 for an explanation of body planes). That image is then used to create an axial image that is tilted through the disk space. This finished product is an image that simulates an axial slice taken with a gantry tilt that matches the angulation of the vertebrae (see Figure 5–4).

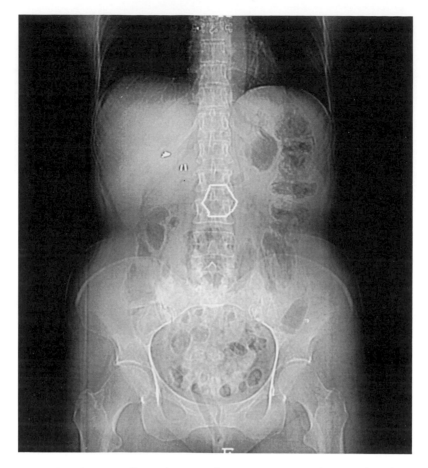

Fig. 5–3.   The correlate function allows the area of aortic aneurysm to be traced on the cross-sectional slices and their outlines to be projected onto the scout image.

In general, the thinner the original slice, the better the reformatted image. Using overlapping slices also improves a reformatted image. Spiral data may be retrospectively reconstructed to create overlapping images for use in reformations. Reformatting is done from image data, and it does not require any changes in scanning parameters. Although image reformatting is useful and often provides additional information, the images produced are not as high quality as actually scanning in another plane.

Three-Dimensional Reformation

The addition of special software allows another type of reformat to be performed. The individual slices are combined and smoothed so that their merged surfaces resemble the intact patient structure. This feature is called **three-dimensional reformation.**

The most common indications for three-dimensional reformations are trauma, tumor, and birth defects. Three-dimensional image generation often plays a vital role in orthopedic and reconstructive surgical planning.

The principles of multiplanar reformation apply to three-dimensional reformats, especially the axiom that the thinner the original CT slices, the better the final three-dimensional image.

A variety of three-dimensional scanning protocols are employed to accommodate the size differences in examination areas. When small structures (e.g., calcaneus, spine, ankle) are examined, it may be best to use a 1.5-mm table increment (spacing) with a 1.5-mm slice thickness. Medium structures (e.g., knee, hip joint, facial bones) typically require a 3-mm table increment with a 3-mm slice thickness.

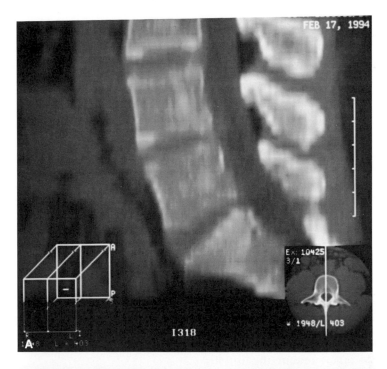

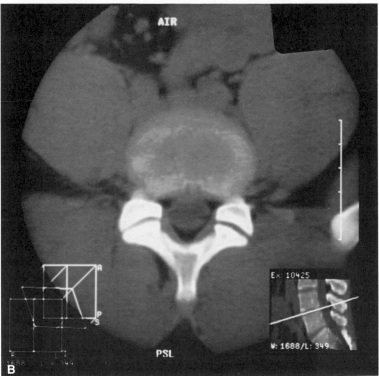

Fig. 5–4. (A) Sagittal reformation of the third to fifth lumbar vertebrae. The image in the lower right shows the reformation plane as it relates to an axial slice. (B) The sagittal reformation was used as the reference image, and an axial reformation, with angulation through the disk space, was created. This axial reformation mimics an image taken with a gantry tilt adjusted for the disk space.

Larger structures (e.g., pelvis) can be scanned with a 4- or 5-mm increment and a 5-mm slice thickness.

Most three-dimensional software programs allow for different combinations of slice spacing and slice thickness within a single three-dimensional model. Consequently, a scanning protocol of thin slices and spacing through the area of primary interest (i.e., fracture or tumor site) could be followed by thicker slices and spacing through the remaining structures. Again, all slices must be contiguous, with no change in gantry tilt, table height, and field of view, and no patient motion during the scanning sequence.

It may be advisable when first creating three-dimensional images to perform several CT scans of a phantom using a variety of scanning techniques. This practice will help to determine the optimal scanning protocol and algorithm for a specific department. Some three-dimensional programs require the image data to be reconstructed in a standard algorithm, whereas others require the use of a bone algorithm.

Usually, it is not necessary to increase the milliampere-second or kilovolt-peak setting on the original study to produce acceptable three-dimensional images. On the contrary, when a scan is performed exclusively for the production of three-dimensional image models, scanning parameters may be decreased.

To create three-dimensional images, a CT department must add a three-dimensional software package to their current CT scanner or obtain a stand-alone three-dimensional computer workstation. Most manufacturers offer a three-dimensional program that is compatible with their system. In addition, several independent firms offer three-dimensional programs that can be used in conjunction with any type of scanner. Some three-dimensional programs allow the use of magnetic resonance imaging (MRI) data as well as CT data.

Three-dimensional imaging offers the technologist the ability to create diagnostic images not obtainable with other imaging modalities. For example, it may not be practical to manipulate a trauma patient to permit a better view of the fractured bone because movement may cause additional trauma to the patient. However, after a CT scan, the three-dimensional image of the fractured bone can be rotated to show the radiologist or surgeon all aspects of the trauma site. In addition, a specific bone can be disarticulated (isolated) and viewed, thus preventing nearby structures from obscuring crucial information about the injury. This imaging capability is also beneficial for patients with tumors and birth defects.

The capabilities of three-dimensional computers and software programs will advance as additional sophisticated imaging technologies are developed. Current and future three-dimensional imaging methods, such as translucent images, cut-plane and melt-through capabilities, two- and three-dimensional cross-reference displays, and three-dimensional measurements, will continue to help to display and analyze hidden and complex structures.

It is important to distinguish reformation from reconstruction. As previously explained, reconstruction uses the originally acquired raw data to form new images. In contrast, reformation, whether it is multiplanar or three-dimensional, uses only image data (see Figure 5-5).

CHAPTER SUMMARY

Changing the window width broadens or narrows the range of visible CT numbers. Window width and window level determine which aspects of an image are visualized. The shades of gray displayed on an image are called the gray scale. The shade of gray that is assigned to a specific anatomic structure is related to the structure's beam attenuation. Higher Hounsfield values are represented by lighter shades of gray. The window width selects the range of Hounsfield units for a particular image, and the window level determines the center Hounsfield unit in this range. In general, the window level is set at roughly the same level as the Hounsfield value of the tissue of interest. Optimal window settings are highly objective, and they vary dramatically within the field. Published window widths and centers are intended to serve as guidelines only. Patient conditions as well as personal preference make considerable adjustments necessary.

Most systems allow the image to be manipulated to facilitate diagnosis. It is important to understand the features available with any given system. Knowing the strengths and weaknesses of specific features will help to

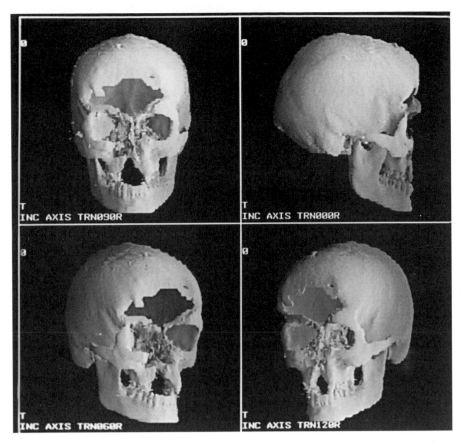

INC AXIS TRN090R

INC AXIS TRN000R

INC AXIS TRN060R

INC AXIS TRN120R

Fig. 5–5. Three-dimensional image showing a gunshot wound to the face.

determine their proper application. The operator's manual published by each manufacturer provides an excellent source of this type of information.

Image magnification may improve lesion detectability by enlarging areas of interest. However, because there is some distortion inherent in the magnification process, it should not be used to replace correct field size selection.

Defining an ROI is the first step in many measurement and display functions. Using a cursor to obtain a Hounsfield measurement furnishes only the measure of one pixel. Selecting an ROI allows an average measurement for all of the pixels within the prescribed region.

Distance measurements provide an estimate of the size of the abnormality. These measurements are also essential in biopsy or drainage procedures. Distance scales alongside the image allow measurements to be taken with calipers.

In many systems, the data are acquired more rapidly than they can be made into images. The data waiting for image reconstruction may often be prioritized to aid in department throughput. This option is not available on all systems.

It is important to annotate images with any information that may not be immediately apparent. Examples of such annotations include: "Images in this study have been flipped, top to bottom" and "Delayed image: 15 minutes post contrast injection."

A variety of names refer to the process of representing each slice in a study on the initial scout image. This cross-referencing is considered standard operating procedure on all CT studies.

Advanced display functions are not routinely used, but they can provide much additional information. Understanding which applications are best suited to each function will aid in diagnosis.

Image reformation requires only the image

data, not the raw data. Certain criteria must be met, however. Images must possess the same image center, display field, and gantry tilt. In addition to these parameters, the images must be contiguous (no missing slices). On the whole, thinner slices produce better reformatted images. Overlapping slices may also improve reformation quality.

REVIEW QUESTIONS

1. Why is a gray scale necessary to display CT images?
2. What does the window width determine?
3. What happens to pixel values that are higher or lower than the range selected by the window width?
4. Provide an example of an area of anatomy that is best imaged with a wide window width. What is an area that is best visualized by a narrow width?
5. What does window level select?
6. When is it helpful to magnify a CT image?
7. What does a high standard deviation indicate?
8. Which factors must be identical if images are to be reformatted?
9. Provide three indications for a three-dimensional reformation.

Chapter 6

RADIATION DOSIMETRY

IONIZING RADIATION

Some forms of energy, such as x-ray radiation, penetrate materials and are absorbed by or cause changes in the material. Usually, the radiation ceases to exist because it transfers its energy to the material that it penetrates. An x-ray can indirectly produce ion pairs in tissue as it transfers energy along its path into the body. The ion pairs react with other chemical systems and cause damage. X-rays may also directly cause damage by striking and breaking molecular bonds, such as those in DNA.

The ionizing radiation used in CT is the x-ray, with maximum energy from 120 to 140 keV and average energy near 70 keV. Radiation exposure results when x-rays pass through matter (air). The unit of exposure is the **roentgen (R),** which is defined as the amount of x- or gamma-ray energy required to produce an electrostatic charge of 0.000258 coulomb (C) in 1 kg air. This unit applies only for exposure to air.

When the x-rays from a CT scanner strike a patient and interact with tissue, most of the energy is absorbed and some of it passes through to the detectors. The unit of absorbed dose is the **rad,** which is equal to the absorption of 0.01 joule (J) of energy per gram of matter. The System Internationale (SI) unit of absorbed dose is the gray (Gy). There are 100 rads in 1 Gy. A centigray (cGy) equals 1 rad. A conversion factor is required to compute rads in tissue from roentgens in air. The factor is nearly 1.0 for diagnostic x-rays and most people ignore the difference.

In recognition of the health effects of x-ray dose, another conversion factor, called the **quality factor (Q),** is applied to absorbed dose to account for the different health effects produced from different types of ionizing radiations. This value for diagnostic x-rays is 1.0, and the unit for dose equivalent is the **rem,** or **radiation equivalent man.** The SI unit for dose equivalent is the **Sievert (Sv).**

There are 100 rem in 1 Sv. This term is used for radiation protection purposes and is usually discussed only for occupational exposure of CT staff.

PATIENT DOSE

The dose to patients is reported in rads or centigray, and results from the absorption of energy from the x-ray beam. Figure 6-1 shows the transaxial radiation slice generated from one tube rotation.

Figure 6-2 shows the ideal radiation profile across a 10-mm slice with no scattered radiation. Because there is scatter in the patient, some of the radiation spreads to tissue outside the designated slice (Figure 6-3).

Most clinical applications of CT involve the use of multiple scans with adjacent or overlapping slices. The effect on the radiation dose to the patient from multiple scans is the addition of the scatter overlap, or tails, of each slice to the central slice radiation dose of neighboring slices (Figure 6-4). When there is no overlap or gap between the slices, the **multiple scan average dose (MSAD)** equals the **CT dose index (CTDI).** The CTDI is reported by manufacturers to the United States Food and Drug Administration (FDA) and to prospective customers regarding the doses typically delivered by their machines.[1] The dose to plastic (Lucite) phantoms is actually reported. The conversion factor (f) for dose in rads from roentgens is 0.78 for Lucite. The dose to tissue (muscle) is more because the f factor is approximately 0.93 at CT energies. If there is slice overlap or gap, the CTDI is multiplied by the ratio of the slice thickness to the slice increment. This value is the MSAD for that technique.

Because of the isocentric rotational nature of the exposure geometry, the center of the patient receives nearly as much radiation as the periphery. Dose uniformity usually applies to head scans, but it decreases as scan field of view and patient size increase (Figure

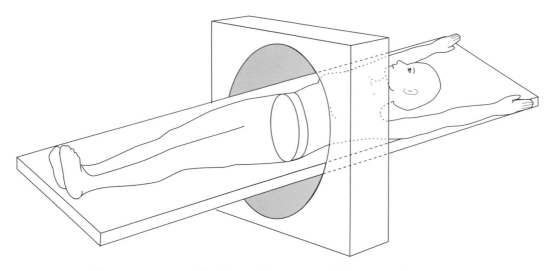

Fig. 6-1. Transaxial radiation slice generated from one tube rotation.

6-5). The central dose for a typical body scan (35-cm thick) is usually one-fifth to one-third the peripheral dose.

In conventional film/screen radiography, the skin of the entrance plane receives the most radiation (100%). The percentage decreases quickly as the x-ray beam penetrates tissue. The exit exposure can be 0.1% to 1% of the entrance exposure (Figure 6-6).

Measurements are usually taken at the center of the slice and at several points around the periphery. Plastic phantoms are used to simulate a patient. The CTDI doses are then reported for typical head and body imaging techniques. These are the radiation doses that a patient receives if multiple scans or contiguous slices are taken. If there is slice overlap or if gaps occur between slices, the CTDI is

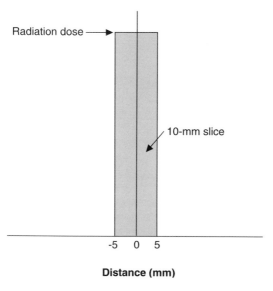

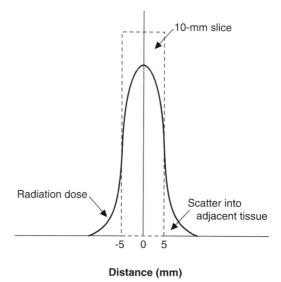

Fig. 6-2. Ideal radiation profile across a 10-mm slice without scattered radiation.

Fig. 6-3. Radiation spreads to tissue outside the designated slice because of scatter in the patient.

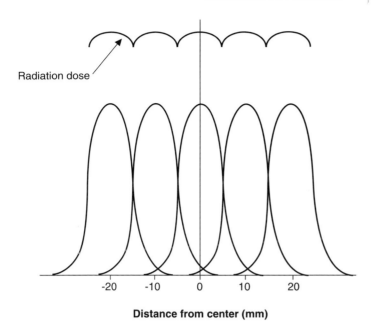

Fig. 6–4. The radiation dose from multiple scans adds scatter overlap from each neighboring slice to the radiation dose of the central slice.

multiplied by the ratio of slice thickness to slice increment. A slice thickness of 10 mm with an 8-mm slice spacing results in an increase in the CTDI of 10:8, or 1.25. This value is technically the MSAD because the CTDI conditions no longer exist.

Measurements may show nonuniform dose levels throughout the phantom from scanners or techniques that have partial or overscan capabilities. In abdominal scans, the peripheral dose usually decreases near the tabletop because of the additional attenuation from the table.

Several factors affect the patient dose from CT. It is important to understand that a simple comparison between doses delivered from CT and from film/screen radiography cannot be conducted. These two imaging modalities

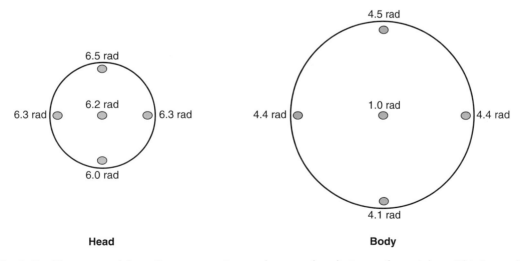

Fig. 6–5. The center of the patient can receive nearly as much radiation as the periphery. This is usually true for head scans; however, it decreases as the scan field of view and patient thickness increase.

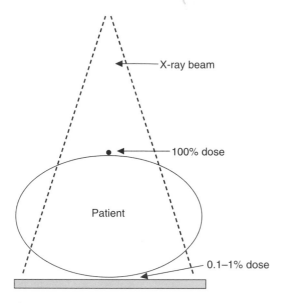

Fig. 6–6. In conventional film/screen radiography, the skin of the entrance plane receives the most radiation (100%). The percentage decreases quickly as the x-ray beam penetrates tissue. The exit exposure can be 0.1% to 1% of the entrance exposure.

are significantly different in principle and purpose and also have different imaging requirements.

Screen/film radiography has good spatial high-contrast resolution or detail capabilities. A standard film/screen system may be able to differentiate, or resolve, a high-contrast pattern (e.g., bone fragments, hairline fractures) up to 15 line pairs per millimeter (lp/mm). Film alone can resolve up to 100 lp/mm. A high-speed system can resolve 6 to 8 lp/mm. A good fluoroscope can resolve 2 to 4 lp/mm. Ultrasound, magnetic resonance imaging (MRI), and CT perform poorly in this category and can resolve only 1 to 2 lp/mm (10–20 lp/cm).

CT is an excellent low-contrast discriminator because of detector dynamics and the precision in calculating the linear attenuation of each pixel. Film/screen systems have much lower low-contrast sensitivity. They typically cannot discriminate objects that have less than 10% contrast with their background material. However, CT can usually resolve and display visual differences between small objects (1–3 mm) that have only minimal difference in density (0.1%–0.5%). This capability

allows visualization of soft tissue masses that are not seen with film/screen systems.

There is a price to be paid to produce good low-contrast images. Image noise must be controlled to allow visualization and diagnosis. The most significant way to suppress the quantum noise in the image is to increase the number of image-carrying quanta (x-ray photons). This change requires an increase in milliampere-seconds (mAs) and an increase in radiation dose. A certain radiation dose (photons per pixel) must be provided to maintain image noise at an acceptable level (1% or less). As a result, the radiation doses for CT examinations are substantially higher than those for film/screen studies of the same body part.

For example, a series of contiguous CT slices of the abdomen typically delivers 2 to 5 rads to the periphery (1–2 rads in the center). An anteroposterior film of the abdomen may produce 0.3 to 0.6 rad at the surface, 0.03 to 0.1 rad in the center, and little radiation at the exit surface (0.002–0.01 rad). If the film is repeated, the dose is multiplied by the number of repetitions with the same technique. There is little likelihood of repeated CT studies for technical reasons, although contrast studies are routinely taken in addition to noncontrast studies, and this practice may double the patient dose.

Angiography and interventional radiography are special procedures that produce radiation doses near or exceeding those from CT. As an example, for cerebral angiography, a series of 10 to 20 films may be taken several times as contrast material is injected into different vessels. The skin dose per film may be 100 to 200 mrads and may decrease rapidly as tissue depth increases. The total skin dose may be 1000 to 10,000 mrads. The average dose to the head is much lower because the exit dose is a fraction of the entrance dose.

Interventional radiography with long fluoroscopic times also produces high radiation exposure to patients. Patients who require several hours of fluoroscopy may have skin exposure of hundreds of roentgens.

FACTORS AFFECTING PATIENT RADIATION DOSE

Scanner Type (Generation)

The x-ray tube is closer to the patient in a fourth-generation scanner than in a third-generation scanner because it spins inside the detector bank circle. This proximity increases skin dose slightly (inverse square law).

Another factor that contributes to an increased dose with a fourth-generation scanner is the requirement for additional radiation to compensate for the scatter radiation accepted at all angles. Because all of the detectors face the patient, scatter radiation can reach these detectors and contribute to noise or image degradation. However, if the detectors are not used to collect data unless the primary beam strikes them, then the dose increase may be less.

Rotation Angle

Theoretically, a rotation arc of only 180° is required to satisfy most reconstruction algorithms. Most scanners employ 360° acquisition angles to compensate for radiation beam divergence and patient motion. The extra scanning information improves image quality, but increases radiation dose. Additionally, overscanning (more than 360°) may be employed to collect more data and improve image quality. Some radiation may also be produced during the overscan as the tube is accelerating or decelerating without data collection.

For rotation arcs other than 360°, the radiation dose to the patient is not uniformly distributed around the slice. For tissue areas that receive the overlap from overscanning, the radiation dose can be significantly higher than that for other parts of the slice. Usually, the location of the overlap cannot be characterized with slip-ring scanners because they do not start and stop the exposure in the same location repeatedly. Some fast scan or partial scan techniques deliver a typical radiation dose to only half of the slice, whereas the half of the slice that does not receive the leading edge of the x-ray beam has a substantially lower dose. Again, it is difficult to characterize the distribution of dose for slip-ring systems.

Radiographic Technique

The tube potential (kilovoltage or kVp) controls the maximum energy of the x-ray beams produced. Typically, scanners operate at 120 to 140 kVp, producing an x-ray spectrum with an average photon energy of approximately 70 keV. The operator usually does not change the kVp setting because many systems have automatic technique protocols for different applications. The kVp setting affects radiographic contrast and dose. As the setting is increased, the radiographic contrast decreases and dose increases if no other changes are made. The ability of the x-ray beam to penetrate tissue also increases, and the ratio of the dose in the center of the slice to the dose at the skin surface increases.

The tube current (mA) controls the rate at which x-rays are produced. The scan time (s or seconds) controls the duration of exposure. Combined, the mAs controls the total number of x-rays produced. There is a linear relationship between the mAs and the radiation dose. If the mAs is doubled, the total dose doubles. However, the dose in a particular region may change, as mentioned previously, for scans less than or greater than 360°. Some scanners employ pulsed x-ray beams in which the x-ray exposure is on for a short period of time to collect data, the beam stops briefly for several technical reasons, and the cycle is repeated many times during each scan. For these systems, the indicated scan time may not reflect the actual exposure time, which is less.

Filtration

Filtration is required to remove some of the soft, or low-energy, x-rays from the beam. These low-energy x-rays would be quickly absorbed by the patient. Photons are needed to penetrate the patient and strike the detectors, but some of them must be absorbed to produce radiographic contrast. Adding metal filters to the beam permits selective removal of x-rays with low energy and reduces the radiation dose while maintaining contrast at an acceptable level. The minimum amount of filtration must be 2.5 mm of aluminum-equivalent material for machines that operate above 90 kVp.[2]

Most systems have additional filtration or compensating filters that are used to help to shape the intensity profile of the x-ray beam. Early head scanners required the use of a water bath around the head to minimize the range of photon intensities striking the detectors. The use of a compensating filter, such as a bow tie filter (thick at the edges, thin in the center), reduces the intensity at the edges of the beam, where the patient is thinnest. As the filtration is increased, patie.... ...creases unless the radiographic technique is increased.

Collimation

Leaded collimators are used near the x-ray tube to control the size of the beam striking the patient. If the radiation beam is not controlled to match the detector size, then there would be additional scatter radiation to degrade the image and produce excessive radiation dose to the patient. Typically, the radiation beam width equals the width of the isocenter (center of gantry).

Collimators may also be used near the detectors for scatter rejection and aperture use. Scatter is rejected like a grid. By closing down the collimators further, more photons are needed, improving image quality through noise reduction, but increasing radiation dose.

Detector Efficiency

Solid-state detectors typically have high efficiency (90%–100%) and require the least amount of radiation exposure. These detectors are commonly used in third- and fourth-generation scanners.

Pressurized-gas detectors, such as xenon, typically are less efficient (50%–60%) and require more radiation dose for the same image statistics.

Scan Field Diameter

The **scan field diameter** is the diameter of the actual irradiated field. The **field of view** is the diameter of the reconstructed and displayed field. If the displayed field is smaller than the scanned field, the area outside the displayed field of view is still irradiated, but with no image information. Larger fields irradiate more tissue and allow more potential scatter to degrade the image. However, for the same radiographic technique (kVp and mAs), a smaller scan field often produces higher radiation doses than a large field because of the greater concentration of radiation from the rotation of the x-ray beam focused on a smaller volume of tissue. Absorbed dose is volume dependent (energy per volume). For example, a head scan with a field of view of 240 to 250 mm may have a surface dose that is 1.5 to 2 times as great as that from

...with a field of view of 350 to 400 mm using the same technique. The total amount of energy deposited in the tissue may be the same, but it is more concentrated with a smaller scan field diameter.

Slice Thickness and Spacing

As slice thickness increases, the volume of tissue irradiated increases and the dose may increase slightly in the slice. However, for multiple-slice examinations, decreasing slice thickness and using contiguous slices will increase the MSAD because of the increased amount of scatter radiation to adjacent slices. Also, to maintain image quality (noise) at the same level, additional radiation is needed for thinner slices.

For multiple-slice examinations with non-contiguous slices, the MSAD changes by the ratio of the slice thickness divided by the slice spacing.

Patient Size

Large patients or thick body parts often require radiographic techniques that increase the radiation dose.

Repeat Scans

Areas of the patient that are rescanned for contrast studies or other technical or clinical reasons receive additional radiation. The effect is cumulative.

Image Matrix Size

Commonly used matrix sizes are 512×512 pixels and 1024×1024 pixels. Increasing the matrix size from 512 to 1024 quadruples the number of pixels in the matrix and increases the spatial resolution capabilities, but requires additional radiation dose to maintain the same statistics in each pixel.

Spiral Technique

With a spiral technique and a pitch of $1:1$, there is no difference in radiation dose relative to axial techniques. A pitch greater than $1:1$ reduces the MSAD, but does not image all of the tissue in that volume. A pitch less than $1:1$ increases the MSAD to the patient.

Localization Scans

Localization scans are called by various names. These scans are digital image acquisitions that are made as the tube is stationary and the table moves through the scan field. The radiation dose for these scanned slit projection radiography techniques is low, on the order of 25 to 100 mrad.

Reconstruction Filters

Reconstruction filters do not affect the radiation dose to the patient unless they change the radiographic technique. Many scanners allow postprocessing of the raw data with different mathematic filters to enhance specific aspects of the image.

RELATIONSHIP BETWEEN DOSE AND IMAGE QUALITY

Image noise is the undesirable fluctuation of pixel values in an image of homogeneous material. It is caused by the combination of many features, the most prevalent being **quantum noise,** or **quantum mottle.** Quantum mottle is inversely related to the number of photons used to form the image. As the number of x-ray photons decreases, noise increases. This effect is represented as:

$$\text{Noise}_{SD} \; \alpha \; \frac{1}{\sqrt{(B \cdot D \cdot h \cdot w^3)}}$$

Noise [standard deviation (SD)] is inversely proportional to the square root of the product of B (beam transmission through the patient), D (maximum surface dose), h (slice thickness), and w cubed (reconstructed pixel width).[3]

Another way to represent this formula is:

$$\text{Dose} \; \alpha \; \frac{1}{[(B)(SD^2)(h)(w^3)]}$$

Dose is inversely proportional to the product of B (beam transmission through patient), SD squared (standard deviation of pixel values), h (slice thickness), and w cubed (reconstructed pixel width).

From a scan of homogeneous material, such as water, the mean CT number and standard deviation can be analyzed using the region of interest (ROI) function. The displayed values indicate how much the CT numbers fluctuate from the average value. An increase in the standard deviation indicates that the value of the CT number of each pixel in the image is increasingly different from the average value in the image noise.

The smaller the noise standard deviation, the smoother the image and the better the low-contrast resolution capability. Spatial resolution can be increased with a smaller pixel width (w), but a 2× decrease in pixel width requires an increase in dose of 8× to maintain the noise at an acceptable level. Spatial resolution in the Z axis can also be increased with a smaller slice width (h); however, a 2× increase in dose is required if the slice width is cut in half to maintain constant noise.

As the patient thickness increases, fractional beam transmission (B) decreases because more of the x-ray beam is absorbed, increasing patient dose.

CHAPTER SUMMARY

The CT image is created using x-ray radiation. The internationally accepted unit of dose is the gray. Another unit that is still often used is the rad. The x-ray energy emitted from the CT tube either is absorbed by the patient or passes through the patient to strike the detector. The dose to the patient is reported in either rads or centigray.

If there were no scatter radiation, the dose of an entire CT study would equal that of a single slice, assuming that each section is exposed only once. Because there is scatter from adjacent slices, the dose for a multiple-slice scan is higher than that for a single slice. Because most CT examinations are done with multiple scans, the dose is calculated with the MSAD. The CTDI is a similar measurement, but it does not take into account protocols that consist of overlapping slices or gaps between slices. The CTDI is what manufacturers report to the FDA and to customers regarding the typical dose for a specific scanner.

In conventional radiography, the skin receives the most radiation and the dose decreases quickly as the beam penetrates the body. In CT, because the x-ray tube travels around the patient, the center of the patient receives nearly as much radiation as the periphery.

Because of the many differences between film/screen radiography and CT, simple comparisons of dose cannot be made. The dose delivered from a CT study is significantly higher than that received from a conventional x-ray study.

Many factors influence the dose received by the patient: scanner type, rotational angle, radiographic technique, filtration, collimation, detector efficiency, scan field diameter, slice thickness and spacing, patient size, repeat scans, and image matrix size.

Radiation dose directly affects image quality. If an insufficient dose is employed in scanning, image noise may become substantial.

REVIEW QUESTIONS

1. How does an x-ray beam damage tissue?
2. What unit is used to report the dose to the patient?
3. What is the quality factor?
4. Why is dose generally calculated with the MSAD rather than a single slice?
5. Explain the difference between MSAD and CTDI.
6. How is conventional radiography superior to CT?
7. What is the disadvantage of producing an image with good low-contrast detectability?
8. What modality exposes the patient to a radiation dose that is similar to that of CT?
9. Explain the effect that an increase in kVp has on the radiation dose to the patient, assuming that all other factors remain the same.
10. How does scan field size affect patient radiation exposure?
11. How is radiation dose related to image quality?

REFERENCES

1. Title 21, Code of Federal Regulations, Part 1020.33.
2. Title 21, Code of Federal Regulations, Part 1020.30(m).
3. Pentlow KS: Dosimetry in computed tomography. In *Radiology of the Skull and Brain: Technical Aspects of Computed Tomography,* vol 5. Edited by Newton TH, Potts DG. St. Louis, CV Mosby, 1981.

Chapter 7

ENHANCEMENT TECHNIQUES

Enhancement techniques typically used in CT fall into the two main categories of intravascular and gastrointestinal. In each category, there is considerable difference of opinion as to optimal dose, rate, and type of contrast. New enhancement techniques continue to be evaluated, with guidelines changing almost monthly. This chapter discusses general scanning principles.

INTRAVASCULAR CONTRAST MATERIALS

Radiographic contrast material increases the ability of the enhanced structure to attenuate the x-ray beam. The iodine atoms in the contrast material are responsible for this increase in attenuation. These beam attenuation abilities are directly related to the concentration of iodine. Abnormal tissue has different contrast enhancement patterns compared with normal tissue. Therefore, intravenous contrast medium is often used to increase the difference in density between a lesion and the normal organ parenchyma.

The concentration of iodine may appear differently depending on manufacturer. The concentration of iodine in solution may be listed as milligrams of iodine per milliliter of solution (generally for low-osmolality agents). Concentration may also be described as percent weight per volume (typically high-osmolality agents). Therefore, comparison of contrast agents can be confusing.

Iodinated contrast media vary significantly from other drugs administered intravascularly. The reason for using iodinated agents is not their pharmacologic action, but rather their distribution in and elimination from the body. The difference between contrast media and therapeutic agents is great when dose and delivery are considered. Therapeutic agents are typically given in small quantities and at regular intervals. On the other hand, contrast agents are given rapidly and in large doses.

Most intravascular drugs are nearly isotonic; that is, they have nearly the same number of particles in solution as water. Contrast agents may have up to seven times the number of particles in solution as water. The structural property of a liquid regarding the number of particles in solution compared with water is known as **osmolality.**

In addition to its high osmolality, contrast material is much more viscous than other intravascular agents. **Viscosity** is a physical property that may be described as the thickness or friction of the fluid as it flows. Molecular structure and concentration affect viscosity. The viscosity of the contrast material can be significantly decreased by heating the liquid to body temperature for injection. This process facilitates rapid injection through small-bore needles and angiographic catheters.

High osmolality and viscosity are the most significant characteristics of water-soluble contrast media that cause the hemodynamic, cardiac, and subjective effects of these media. Sudden, drastic transfer of water from the interstitial and cellular spaces into the plasma is caused by osmotic pressure gradients. This change explains many of the adverse effects of contrast agents. These effects include vasodilation, increased heat, pain, various hemodynamic changes, and osmotic diuresis.[1]

Newer contrast agents have lower osmolality than older agents. However, even the new agents have twice the osmolality of blood. These new contrast agents are often referred to as low-osmolar contrast media, and the older agents are called high-osmolar contrast media.

The molecules of intravascular contrast agents may also be classified according to whether they are ionic or nonionic. Ionic contrast medium forms ions in water solutions. Nonionic contrast medium does not dissociate; therefore, it does not ionize in water. Although many nonionic contrast agents also

51

have low osmolality, the two terms are not synonymous. A low-osmolar contrast medium may be ionic, for example, Hexabrix solution.

Product literature often mentions the ratio of iodine atoms to dissolved particles. This information is important because a higher ratio indicates better opacification (more iodine), whereas a lower ratio indicates low osmolality (fewer side effects).

Physiologic Effects

A rapid bolus injection of contrast medium into the venous system causes a rapid increase in the osmolality of the plasma because of the hypertonic contrast material. This increase in plasma osmolality causes a transfer of water from red blood cells and pulmonary tissue into the plasma space in response to a large osmotic gradient. This fluid shift causes a decrease in hematocrit level and an increase in plasma volume. After the hypertonic mixture of blood and contrast material transits the pulmonary vascular system, the osmotic pressure gradient is reversed as blood without contrast material flows into the pulmonary tissue. Thus, water shifts back into the pulmonary tissue. If the initial osmotic stress produces significant endothelial cell shrinkage in the pulmonary capillaries, the intercellular clefts may open and allow proteins to move into the pulmonary interstitial space. These conditions cause additional fluid to accumulate in the lungs.[1]

Renal Clearance

Clearance of contrast agents occurs primarily through renal excretion. In patients with complete kidney failure, elimination of contrast material occurs through the liver and gut. This type of clearance is referred to as vicarious excretion. It occurs at a much slower rate than kidney excretion. Under normal conditions, nearly 100% of the contrast medium is eliminated through the kidneys. Renal clearance is typically described by the term half-time, which is the time required for one-half of the iodine to be cleared. In patients with normal renal function, the half-time is between 1 and 2 hours for all classes of contrast agents.

The peak time for renal excretion of contrast medium is approximately 3 minutes after intravenous injection. Urine iodine concentration peaks approximately 60 minutes after administration. Because of its osmolality, the contrast agent has a diuretic effect, and water and sodium excretion will increase within minutes after injection. In addition to urine, other substances are excreted, including potassium, calcium, phosphorus, magnesium, uric acid, urea, and oxalate. Subsequently, the injection of iodinated contrast material can cause significant patient dehydration.

A risk of renal failure is also associated with the injection of contrast agents. Nephrotoxic effects are usually limited to an asymptomatic transient period of renal dysfunction; however, some patients experience acute renal failure requiring dialysis, and, in rare instances, patients die.[2]

The likelihood of severe renal complications as a result of contrast injection is small. However, several risk factors increase the chance of nephrotoxicity. They are listed in Table 7-1.

Central Nervous System Involvement

The central nervous system is separated from substances in the blood by the blood–brain barrier. Patients who have diseases that affect the blood–brain barrier may be at increased risk from contrast administration because the contrast material may enter the brain more readily. In the general population, seizures after intravenous contrast medium administration are rare, with an incidence of approximately 0.01%. However, seizures may occur in 6% to 19% of patients with brain metastasis. The risk of seizure development, especially in patients with brain metastasis, may be reduced by intravenous injection of 5 mg diazepam before the injection of contrast medium. Seizures can also be controlled with diazepam.[1]

Table 7-1. Risk Factors in the Development of Contrast-Induced Acute Renal Failure[2]

Preexisting renal insufficiency
Diabetes mellitus
Multiple myeloma
Dehydration
Previous contrast-induced acute renal failure
Advanced age
Vascular disease

Adapted with permission from Humes D: *Radiocontrast-Induced Nephrotoxicity*. Princeton, NJ, Squibb Diagnostics, 1989, p 13.

In neurologic CT scanning, the enhancement of most brain lesions is caused by blood–brain barrier disruption, not the intrinsic vascularity of the tissue. Because modern scanners are so rapid, all of the contrast material should be administered before the start of scanning.[3]

High-Osmolality Versus Low-Osmolality Iodinated Contrast Media

Traditional high-osmolality, ionic contrast agents have been used for more than 30 years and are considered safe and effective. Several adverse reactions are reported, most of them minor. However, some patients have serious reactions that may be life threatening. Prompt and appropriate treatment is critical in these cases. Although this text does not discuss the treatment of acute contrast medium reactions, all personnel involved in scanning should be familiar with the recommended standards of treatment.

Newer contrast agents, called low-osmolar, or nonionic, were introduced in recent years. The reaction rate with these agents is about one-fifth that with conventional ionic contrast agents.[4] Patients experience much less discomfort, nausea, and vomiting when the low-osmolar agents are used. Unfortunately, these newer contrast agents do not eliminate serious reactions, and fatal reactions also occur.[5]

Ideally, the newer agents can be used exclusively. However, because of their high cost compared with standard high-osmolality agents, this practice is not always possible. Therefore, many facilities screen patients for risk factors for adverse reactions to contrast material. These patients are given low-osmolality medium. Table 7–2 lists the guidelines

Table 7–2. Risk Factors for Developing Adverse Reactions to Contrast Media

Previous reaction to contrast material (except flushing, heat, nausea, or vomiting)
History of asthma
Significant allergic history (not to drugs)
Renal or cardiac impairment (including cardiac decompensation, severe arrhythmia, unstable angina, recent myocardial infarction, pulmonary hypertension)
Poor hydration
Diabetes mellitus
Myelomatosis
Sickle-cell anemia
Youth (infants, young children)

developed from the Royal Australian College of Radiology (RACR) Survey of Intravenous Contrast Media Reactions.

In addition to the RACR guidelines, the American College of Radiology suggested in its 1990 report the following risk factors indicating the use of low-osmolality contrast material:

1. Severe generalized debilitation
2. Risk of aspiration
3. Acute anxiety about the contrast procedure
4. Communication problem precluding identification of these risk factors

Regardless of the type of contrast medium used, some reactions will occur. The following methods improve the safety of contrast injection:

1. Do not inject contrast material in an isolated setting. Help should be immediately available, with additional assistance accessible should a full-blown anaphylaxis-like reaction or cardiac arrest occur.
2. Have immediately available the equipment and medication necessary to treat a reaction.
3. Have basic medical knowledge about the patient.
4. Have prior training in the treatment of various types of reactions. Training in cardiopulmonary resuscitation (CPR) is necessary; training in basic life support (BLS) or advanced cardiac life support (ACLS) protocols is recommended.
5. Be able to identify the specific type of reaction so that appropriate, effective treatment can be initiated quickly.
6. Provide early treatment, which permits the use of lower doses of drugs to reverse the reaction, thereby minimizing drug side effects (particularly important with drugs such as epinephrine).[1]

Injection Route

The proximal forearm or a medially placed antecubital vein is the best site for administration of contrast material. The use of peripheral forearm or hand veins must be carefully monitored, and injection rates must be lowered.

Mechanical flow-control contrast injectors have a pressure limit. They attempt to deliver the flow rate that is selected if it does not exceed the pressure limit [measured in pounds per square inch (psi)]. If this pressure rate is reached, injection will continue, but at a slower rate than selected. This feature does not prevent the extravasation of contrast medium into the subcutaneous tissue, however. Therefore, the injection site must be carefully monitored during injection.

Indwelling central lines, such as INFUSE-A-PORT, PORT-A-CATH, and Hickman catheters, are not recommended for contrast injection. Many of these lines have a lower psi rating than standard intravenous catheters. In some patients, central lines are damaged by the rapid injection of contrast material. If possible, a peripheral intravenous line should be started and used for the administration of contrast.

Often, patient conditions preclude the use of peripheral intravenous sites. Using central lines for injecting contrast medium may be the only option in some cases. Because of the lower psi rating of some catheters, certain precautions should be taken. The following guidelines were developed by Swedish Hospital in Seattle, Washington.[6]

1. Use a rate of injection that is no greater than 0.8 ml/sec on central venous catheters and Landmark.
2. Use a 1-inch 18-gauge needle to inject contrast material into the injection cap of the intravenous line.
3. Flush the line with 10 ml normal saline before injection to assess the patency of the line. Use firm, steady pressure, but no force to check line patency.
4. Use only the following central venous catheters: Hickman, PORT-A-CATH, double- and triple-lumen Burron.
5. Do not use any access route that is inflamed or painful.
6. Use a pulmonary artery (Swan-Ganz) catheter only with the proximal or VIP lumens that open into the right atrium. The distal lumen (pulmonary artery) should never be used for contrast administration. These lines must be used exclusively by staff familiar with the various catheter lumens.

7. Notify a physician of any problem with a central venous catheter after contrast injection.

Extravasation

Because of the routine use of intravenous contrast material in the CT department, extravasation of contrast medium into the subcutaneous tissue sometimes occurs. The use of mechanical injectors produces the best results. However, if appropriate precautions are not taken, extravasation is likely to be more common and more severe with the routine use of a power injector. Every effort should be made to avoid contrast extravasation because the results may be serious.

Most injuries involve small volumes and are not clinically significant. Slight swelling and erythema may develop and usually subside without complication. Severe tissue necrosis can be caused by even small-volume (less than 10 ml) extravasation, and surgical intervention may be required.[1]

There is no universally accepted treatment for contrast extravasation. Treatment may include local application of heat for the first 6 hours, then application of cold; local injection of isoproterenol or propranolol; local injection of steroids; and surgical drainage. The results of the various courses of treatment are mixed, and the best method of reducing injury is prevention.

Strict adherence to the following guidelines will substantially reduce the risk of contrast extravasation:

1. Start an intravenous line with a 1.5-inch, 18- to 20-gauge needle with a flexible (plastic) cannula. A needle that is 22 gauge or smaller requires the injection rate to be decreased.
2. Monitor the injection site, preferably a medially directed antecubital vein, during the initial phase of injection. Swelling at the site of injection indicates extravasation, and the injection should be stopped immediately.
3. Warm the contrast medium to body temperature to reduce contrast viscosity.
4. Do not use multiple injections into the same vein.

Recent animal studies show that nonionic contrast medium is less injurious to cutaneous and subcutaneous tissue than conventional high-osmolar contrast material.[7] Recent experience with large-volume extravasations of nonionic contrast material shows resolution in all cases, without treatment and without significant morbidity.[8]

Administration Techniques

Although the usefulness of intravenous contrast agents is universally accepted, there is little agreement as to the best method of administering contrast material.

In abdominal CT, the ability to characterize abnormalities of the liver, spleen, pancreas, and kidneys is significantly improved by the use of intravenous contrast enhancement. In addition, vascular characteristics of abnormal tissue may be assessed. Enhancement also helps in differentiating vessels from masses. Contrast enhancement also defines structures in the retroperitoneum and improves the detection of enlarged lymph nodes in the pelvis. Contrast enhancement in the mediastinum and hilar region more readily delineates disease. Because CT examinations are improved with contrast enhancement, it is used in most examinations.

In some cases, intravenous contrast medium diminishes lesion detectability, such as with certain types of liver metastasis that are hypervascular. These lesions may become isodense (the same density as surrounding tissue) in the equilibrium phase of enhancement. Therefore, if scans cannot be acquired before the equilibrium phase (e.g., with older, slower scanners), these lesions become difficult or impossible to detect if only an enhanced study is performed. For this reason, patients with a history of cancer are often scanned without contrast enhancement through the liver, and the entire abdomen is then scanned with intravenous contrast medium. As scan speed increases, these precontrast studies are becoming less common. The phases of contrast enhancement are discussed in the next section.

In many cases, lesions are detected without the use of intravenous contrast agents. However, in nearly all circumstances, contrast enhancement provides more information.

Effects of Contrast Material on Tissue Enhancement

Three phases of tissue enhancement are commonly discussed in CT: the bolus phase, the nonequilibrium phase, and the equilibrium phase. The difference between these phases is predominantly determined by the rate at which the contrast material is delivered and the time that elapses between injection and scanning. The bolus phase, which immediately follows an intravenous bolus injection, is characterized by an attenuation difference of 30 or more Hounsfield units (HU) between the aorta and the inferior vena cava. In the nonequilibrium phase, which follows the bolus phase, there is a difference of 10 to 30 HU between the aorta and the inferior vena cava. The last phase is the equilibrium phase, in which the attenuation difference is less than 10 HU. Compared with examinations performed before the administration of contrast medium, visualization of tumors in the liver is improved in the nonequilibrium phase, but not in the equilibrium phase. Scanning in the equilibrium phase does not improve visualization of hepatic tumors compared with precontrast examination, and this practice carries a considerable risk of tumor enhancement.[1]

Lesions, particularly hepatic tumors, are most likely to be detected when scans are acquired before the equilibrium phase. Because scanners vary in speed, the degree to which this goal is accomplished will vary accordingly. However, the proper timing of contrast injection can greatly enhance the capability of scanners, both high-end spiral models and less expensive, traditional models. To obtain consistent, reproducible injection results, a mechanical flow-control injector is essential.

Methods of Injection

The two most common methods of administering contrast material are the drip infusion and bolus techniques. In the drip infusion technique, an intravenous line is initiated and contrast medium is allowed to drip in over a period of several minutes. Scanning usually begins after approximately 50 ml of contrast material is injected (roughly 2–3 minutes). The remaining contrast medium continues to drip until administration is complete. This method is not recommended because virtually all of the scans acquired with this technique are taken in the equilibrium phase. Quality significantly diminishes with the use of methods of contrast injection that employ lower doses of contrast material or slower rates of injection. An infusion-type scan is probably the least effective method of abdominal imaging and, in some respects, is even inferior to scanning without contrast enhancement.[9]

The bolus technique of contrast enhancement employs scanning after a rapid injection of contrast material. A volume of contrast of 50 to 100 ml is injected at a rate of 1 to 4 ml/sec shortly before scanning begins. The interval between the initiation of the injection and the start of scanning is critical, particularly in high-speed scanning. The appropriate interval is also debated. If scanning begins 30 seconds after the injection, the liver is seen with all of the contrast material in the arteries (arterial phase). This phase is optimal for visualizing certain metastatic lesions of the liver. However, when scanning begins so soon after injection, the inferior vena cava as well as other vascular structures are unenhanced because the contrast material does not have time to circulate and reach the venous phase. Without the benefit of contrast enhancement, it may be difficult to discern a normal vascular structure from an abnormality such as a hemangioma. For this reason, some institutions suggest scanning through the liver twice, once in the arterial phase and again in the venous phase of enhancement (the first series 30 seconds after contrast injection and the second series approximately 3 minutes after injection). However, because of the increased radiation exposure and film usage and decreased patient throughput, this routine is not widely used. Most radiologists adopt a procedure that begins scanning between 1 and 3 minutes after the start of injection. When clinically indicated, procedures are often modified to permit scanning during the arterial liver phase.

When scanners cannot scan the entire area of interest rapidly, a modification of the bolus technique is used. This method, which is called **dynamic sequential bolus CT,** employs a series of smaller bolus injections given at intervals over the length of the scan procedure.

Another injection protocol used in conjunction with older, slower scanners is biphasic injection. A bolus phase is used to gain peak enhancement, and a slower second phase is used to extend enhancement until the scanner can complete the study.

Injection Techniques for Spiral Scanning

Injection techniques for spiral scanning are still being studied. Several articles discuss injection rates and scan delay, but no protocol is documented as superior overall. In general, because of its increased speed, spiral scanning allows for a single bolus injection. This bolus is achieved with higher flow rates, and it increases the enhancement level for the entire study. Again, the interval between the injection of contrast material and scanning plays a critical role.

CT Portography and CT Angiography

Less commonly used in CT are the enhancement techniques of CT portography and hepatic CT angiography. CT portography requires placement of a catheter tip in the superior mesenteric artery, distal to any hepatic artery branches. For hepatic CT angiography, femoral artery catheterization is performed, and the catheter is placed into the celiac artery. These techniques are discussed in advanced texts.

GASTROINTESTINAL CONTRAST MEDIUM

In the gastrointestinal tract, contrast medium is essential to distinguish a loop of bowel from a cyst, abscess, or neoplasm. For this reason, oral contrast material is used in most CT scans of the abdomen and pelvis. Options available in oral preparations include a barium sulfate solution and a water-soluble agent. The ideal agent should provide adequate differentiation of bowel from surrounding structures without creating artifacts.

Barium Sulfate Solutions

Conventional radiography suspensions cannot be used in CT. Such full-strength solutions would cause too many streak artifacts. These conventional agents cannot simply be diluted for use in CT because of their tendency to settle after ingestion. This tendency leads to irregular opacification of the bowel. Fortunately, products are available specifically for use in CT. These products contain a 1% to 3% barium sulfate suspension and are specially formulated to resist settling.

A higher dose of oral contrast material provides greater bowel opacification. A minimum of 500 ml of dilute barium sulfate should be given 45 minutes to 2 hours before scanning. An additional 200 ml should be given just before scanning to fill the stomach and proximal small bowel.

In patients who cannot take fluids by mouth, a nasogastric tube may be inserted. The contrast medium can be introduced through the tube. If vomiting is a problem, slowing the rate of administration may help.

The typical low-concentration, low-viscosity solutions may not be adequate for an esophageal study. In such cases, the high-viscosity, low-concentration barium pastes designed for this purpose are recommended.

Barium sulfate should not be given if perforation of the gastrointestinal tract is suspected. Barium leaking into the peritoneal cavity is referred to as **barium peritonitis.** The mortality rate from this condition is significant, and complications can be prevented with the use of water-soluble contrast agents.

Barium sulfate is an inert substance that passes through the body basically unchanged. Allergic reactions to oral barium sulfate solutions are rare. The product literature reports severe reactions in approximately 1 in 500,000 cases and fatalities in 1 in 2 million cases. It is likely that these reactions can be attributed to the additives in the suspension (e.g., flavorings). Although procedural complications are rare, they include aspiration pneumonitis, barium impaction, and intravasation.[10]

Although definitive answers are not available, fewer complications from aspiration appear to occur with barium sulfate than with water-soluble agents.

Water-Soluble Agents

Both ionic and nonionic water-soluble contrast agents can be diluted and administered orally. Because of their unpleasant taste, flavoring is normally added to the solution. A 2% to 5% solution of a water-soluble agent is

normally used. Even with these dilute solutions, iodinated contrast agents usually stimulate intestinal peristalsis. Many patients experience diarrhea after the ingestion of water-soluble agents. Dosages are similar to those used with barium sulfate. However, water-soluble oral contrast material tends to pass through the gastrointestinal tract slightly faster.

It has been traditionally thought that, given orally, the low-osmolality contrast medium offered no advantages over the less expensive high-osmolality contrast medium. Research with pediatric patients has challenged this belief. Researchers of oral contrast medium in newborns have concluded that low-osmolality contrast medium offers a significant reduction in complications compared with barium sulfate or hyperosmolar water-soluble substances.[11] Low-osmolality contrast agents should be used in infants and young children under the following conditions: (1) when the possibility of entry of contrast agent into the lung exists; or (2) when the possibility of leakage of contrast agent from the gastrointestinal tract exists.[12]

Studies of older children revealed an additional advantage. Since the low-osmolality contrast medium has a neutral taste when diluted, patient cooperation is much greater.[13]

When rectosigmoid abnormality is suspected, rectal administration of contrast material may be necessary. In these cases, 150 to 200 ml of a dilute water-soluble agent (1%–3%) is given by enema.

Barium sulfate and water-soluble contrast material cause comparable bowel opacification. Because of the low concentrations used, neither coats the mucosa significantly. Instead, most visible contrast is attributed to the agents filling the bowel. Barium sulfate, in small amounts, tends to cling to the intestinal wall, providing a minimum of visible contrast. In comparison, a small quantity of water-soluble oral contrast is usually absorbed by the bowel.

CHAPTER SUMMARY

Contrast agents are generally classified as either intravascular or gastrointestinal. Throughout radiology literature, there is enormous variation in what is considered optimal enhancement.

Contrast medium attenuates more of the x-ray beam and is used to differentiate between normal and abnormal tissue.

The characteristics that cause the side effects that are common with iodinated contrast material are high osmolality and viscosity. Heating the contrast material to body temperature reduces the viscosity of the liquid.

Contrast agents are currently available with substantially lower osmolality. Fewer reactions occur when these agents are used. Because of the significantly increased cost of these newer agents, many facilities have guidelines for their use. Unfortunately, the newer contrast agents do not eliminate all reactions, and fatal reactions can still occur with their use. Therefore, it is prudent to take basic precautions whenever intravenous contrast material is administered.

Another characteristic of intravenous contrast agents is their ionic nature. This characteristic is separate from osmolality, but they both relate to the agent's chemical structure.

Iodinated contrast medium is excreted through the kidneys. Peak time for excretion by the kidney is approximately 3 minutes after administration. Contrast injection may lead to dehydration. A risk of renal failure is also associated with the injection of contrast medium. There are nine risk factors that help to predict which patients have the greatest likelihood of nephrotoxic effects.

Patients with brain metastasis have an increased incidence of seizures after the injection of contrast material. Because the enhancement of most brain lesions is caused by interruption of the blood–brain barrier, it is important to allow all of the contrast medium to be administered before scanning begins. To reduce the likelihood of potentially serious contrast extravasation, certain guidelines pertaining to injection site should be followed carefully. Care should be used when injecting into central lines because they may not withstand pressure as well as standard intravenous catheters.

Although much can be learned from an unenhanced CT scan, a contrast-enhanced study provides more information. Mechanical flow-control injectors are recommended for use in body scanning. Drip infusion is the least effective injection method, and its use is strongly discouraged.

Tissue enhancement has three phases: the bolus phase, the nonequilibrium phase, and the equilibrium phase. Optimal lesion detection occurs before the equilibrium phase.

With rapid scanners, contrast timing is especially critical. Radiologists do not agree on the best interval between contrast injection and scanning. Often the technique depends on the suspected lesion.

A modified injection technique is used for slower scanners. This technique requires a series of smaller bolus injections administered over the length of the procedure. Another option for slow scanners is the use of biphasic injection.

Oral contrast agents are important in differentiating a bowel loop from an abnormal fluid collection or mass. Manufacturers offer special low-concentration, low-viscosity agents for use in CT. Barium sulfate suspensions or water-soluble solutions provide adequate bowel opacification. However, barium sulfate suspensions should not be used in patients with suspected gastrointestinal perforation.

REVIEW QUESTIONS

1. Why does contrast material appear as a lighter shade of gray on the CT image?
2. How does the administration of contrast medium differ from that of therapeutic agents?
3. Define isotonic and osmolality.
4. Which two characteristics of intravenous contrast material account for most side effects?
5. How does the temperature of intravenous contrast medium affect injection?
6. What is the difference between ionic and nonionic contrast material?
7. How is contrast medium eliminated from the body?
8. What is the peak time for excretion of contrast medium by the kidney? When does urine iodine concentration peak?
9. Which patients are at high risk for the development of contrast-induced acute renal failure?
10. Which patients are at high risk for seizures after intravenous contrast administration?
11. Why should contrast injection be complete before the brain is scanned?
12. Why are indwelling central lines not recommended for contrast injection?

13. What steps can be taken to avoid contrast extravasation into soft tissue?

14. When may intravenous contrast medium actually impair the detectability of a lesion?

15. What are the three phases of contrast enhancement?

16. Which phase provides the greatest likelihood of lesion detection?

17. Why is the interval between the injection of contrast material and the start of scanning important?

18. When is barium sulfate contraindicated?

REFERENCES

1. Katzberg R: *The Contrast Media Manual.* Baltimore, Williams & Wilkins, 1992, pp 1, 2, 12, 16, 20, 21, 68, 80.

2. Humes D: *Radiocontrast-Induced Nephrotoxicity.* Princeton, NJ, Squibb Diagnostics, 1989, p 2.

3. Mallinckrodt Medical, Inc. *Handbook of Computed Tomography: Techniques & Protocols.* St. Louis, MO, Mallinckrodt Medical, Inc., 1992.

4. McClennan BL, Preston M: Ionic and nonionic iodinated contrast media: Evolution and strategies for use. *American Journal of Radiology* 155:225-233, 1990.

5. Curry NS, Schabel SI, Reiheld CT, et al: Fatal reactions to intravenous nonionic contrast material. *Radiology* 178:361-362, 1991.

6. Use of intravenous catheters for all divisions of medical imaging. Seattle, Swedish Hospital.

7. Cohan RH, Leder RA, Bolick D, et al: Extravascular extravasation of radiographic contrast media. *Invest Radiol* 25:504-510, 1990.

8. Cohan RH, Dunnick NR, Leder RA, Baker ME: Extravasation of nonionic radiologic contrast media: Efficacy of conservative treatment. *Radiology* 176:65-67, 1990.

9. Berland L: *Practical CT: Technology and Techniques.* New York, Raven Press, 1987.

10. E-Z-EM product information. E-Z-EM, Inc., Westbury, NY.

11. Langer R, Kaufman HJ: The use of nonionic contrast medium for gastrointestinal studies in infants. Presented at the 72nd Scientific Assembly and Annual Meeting of the RSNA, Chicago, November 30 to December 6, 1986.

12. Cohen M: Choosing contrast media for the evaluation of the gastrointestinal tract of neonates and infants. *Radiology* 162:447-456, 1987.

13. Smevik B, Westvik J: Iohexol for contrast enhancement of bowel in pediatric abdominal CT. *Acta Radiologica* 31;Fasc. 6:601-603, 1990.

Chapter 8

GENERAL IMAGING TECHNIQUES

This chapter discusses CT scanning principles that are not covered under any of the classifications from previous chapters. These principles are standard practice in most, but not all, CT departments.

IMAGING PLANES

Understanding the intricacies of CT scanning requires familiarity with imaging planes. Body planes can be explained with the bread slicing analogy in Chapter 1. A brief review of the directional terms used in medicine may make a discussion of body planes easier to understand.

All directional terms are based on the body being viewed in the anatomic position. This position is characterized by an individual standing erect, with the palms of the hands facing forward (see Figure 8-1). This position is used internationally and guarantees uniformity in descriptions of direction.

The terms **anterior** and **ventral** refer to movement forward (toward the face). **Posterior** and **dorsal** are equivalent terms used to describe movement toward the back surface of the body.

Inferior refers to movement toward the feet (down) and is synonymous with **caudal** (toward the tail or, in humans, the feet). **Superior** defines movement toward the head (up) and is used interchangeably with the term **cranial. Lateral** refers to movement toward the sides of the body. Inversely, **medial** refers to movement toward the midline of the body.

The terms **distal** and **proximal** are most often used in referring to extremities (limbs). Distal (away from) refers to movement toward the ends. The distal end of the forearm is the end to which the hand is attached. Proximal (close to), which is the opposite of distal, may be defined as situated near the point of attachment. For example, the proximal end of the arm is the end at which it attaches to the shoulder.

To help to visualize the imaginary body planes, it is helpful to think of large sheets of glass cutting through the body in various ways. All sheets of glass that are parallel to the floor are called **horizontal,** or **transverse,** planes. Those that stand perpendicular to the floor are called **vertical,** or **longitudinal,** planes (see Figure 8-2).

A sheet of glass that divides the body into anterior and posterior sections is the **coronal** plane. The **sagittal** plane divides the body into right and left sections. The sagittal plane that is located directly in the center, making left and right sections of equal size, is appropriately referred to as the **median,** or **midsagittal,** plane. A **parasagittal** plane is located to either the left or the right of the midline. **Axial** planes are cross-sectional planes that divide the body into upper and lower sections. **Oblique** planes are sheets of glass that are slanted and lie at an angle to one of the three standard planes (see Figure 8-3).

Changing the image plane shows the same structures in a new perspective. The loaf of bread analogy can help to explain this change. For example, if a coin is baked within the bread and lies standing on edge in the loaf, a sharp knife cutting through the bread lengthwise will show the coin as a flat, rectangular density. However, if the bread is restacked and cut in an axial plane, the coin appears circular (see Figure 8-4).

The image plane can be adjusted by positioning the patient, gantry, or both to permit scanning in the desired plane or by reformatting the image data (see Chapter 5). Scanning in the desired plane produces better images than reformatting existing data.

Changing imaging planes in CT provides additional information in a fashion similar to the coin within the bread. Changing the imaging plane from axial to coronal is indicated for two distinct reasons. The primary reason is when the anatomy lies vertically rather than

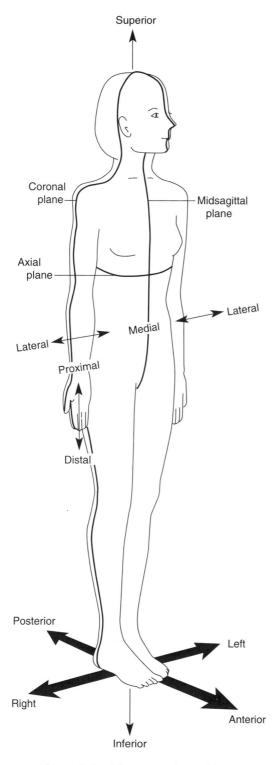

Figure 8-1. The anatomic position.

horizontally. The ethmoid sinuses are an example of this principle. Because the ethmoid turbinates lie predominately in the vertical plane, images taken in an axial plane show only sections of the anatomy, with no view of the entire ethmoid complex (see Figure 8-5A). In Figure 8-5B, the images are taken in the coronal plane, which is more suitable for displaying the ethmoid sinus structures and more readily shows an obstruction.

In the case of the sinus, it is relatively easy to change the patient's position so that images can be acquired coronally. Obviously, this practice is not possible with all areas of the anatomy that may benefit from coronal imaging, for example, the pelvis. Because fat planes in the pelvis often run obliquely or parallel to the transverse plane, in some cases, images obtained in the coronal plane may be superior to those obtained in the axial plane.* However, scanning in the coronal plane is not common because of the difficulty of positioning the pelvis. In this case, reformatting image data into a coronal plane may be useful.

The second indication for scanning in a different plane is to reduce artifacts created by surrounding structures. For this reason, the coronal plane is preferred for scanning the pituitary gland. In the axial plane, the number of streak artifacts and the partial volume effect are greater than in the coronal plane. (See the pituitary protocol in Chapter 9.)

Most scans are performed in the axial plane, but many head protocols require coronal scans.

There are two methods of achieving a coronal position for head scanning. One is to place the patient prone (belly down) on the scanning table and ask the patient to extend the chin forward. An alternative approach is to place the patient supine (belly up) and ask him to drop his head back as far as possible. This position usually requires a specialized head holder. In either position, the slice plane will be coronal. If the patient cannot extend the neck fully, the gantry may be angled to obtain a more coronal plane. The image obtained in either the prone or the supine coronal position is essentially the same. Obviously, the images are flipped inferior-superior. The preferred position involves several factors, including patient comfort, radiologist preference, and the effect of gravity on anatomic

---

* Optimal separation of adjacent structures occurs when the fat plane is perpendicular to the imaging plane.

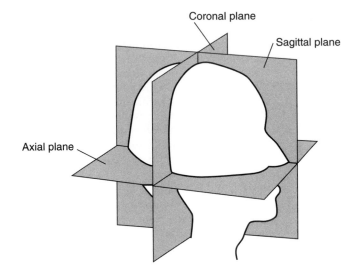

Figure 8–2. Imaging planes.

structures (e.g., will fluid settle inferiorly or superiorly?).

ROUTINE SCANNING PROCEDURES

The following chapters provide general guidelines in a tabular format to facilitate easy reference. Although in actual scanning, there are exceptions to every rule, some standards of practice are assumed. This section discusses these assumptions.

In all routine studies, a digital x-ray image, or scout, is acquired before scanning. The optimal scout includes all areas to be scanned and therefore ensures that the anatomy to be imaged is within the range of the system. A patient may lie out of the scannable range if she is positioned too close to the end of the scanning table.

Regardless of the type of scanner used, it is imperative that the operator input the correct directional instructions before scanning. This procedure requires indicating whether the patient is placed head or feet first into the gantry and whether he is lying supine, prone, or in the decubitus position. If the operator accurately enters this information into the system, the software correctly annotates the image as to left–right and anterior–posterior orientation.

After the scout image is obtained, the operator selects the location of cross-sectional slices. Most scan procedures rely on beginning and ending landmarks that can be seen on the scout image. For example, an abdomen study typically begins at the level of the right diaphragm and terminates at the level of the iliac crest. Both the diaphragm and the iliac crest are easily identifiable on the scout image. With some protocols, it is impossible to use readily identifiable landmarks. In these cases, the operator must make an educated guess, take one image to check the accuracy of the guess, and then proceed. This procedure is often helpful when scanning the adrenal gland. In this situation, a thin slice is required at the level of the adrenals. However, from the scout image, there is no way to predict with any degree of accuracy where the adrenals lie within the abdomen. Obviously, checking the first image before proceeding

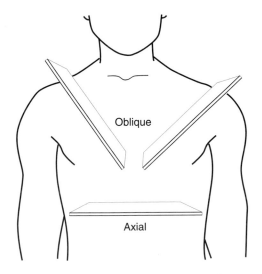

Figure 8–3. Oblique planes lie at an angle to one of the standard planes.

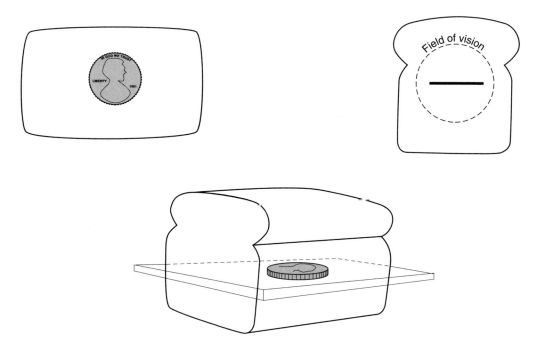

Figure 8–4. The imaging plane will affect the way that an area of anatomy is represented on the cross-sectional slice.

slows down the examination process, but the delay is unavoidable.

It is important to correctly annotate the image as to whether contrast material is administered. All CT systems allow a notation concerning contrast. Often, the notation +C is added after the introduction of contrast medium.

Careful breathing instructions should be given to all patients undergoing body scanning. Some manufacturers suggest that technologists use a coaching procedure to increase the length of breath hold for a spiral study. This coaching requires the patient to take several deep breaths before taking one final breath and holding it for the maximum possible time, then exhaling slowly.

After completion of a study, it is standard procedure to include a scout image that is cross-referenced by lines. These lines represent the location of each cross-sectional image. It is also typical to include patient data at the end of each examination.

Routine procedure for many CT examinations includes scanning without contrast material, then repeating the study with intravenous contrast enhancement. Whenever possible, the repeat scans should be taken at the same location as the unenhanced images. Comparing the slice with and without contrast enhancement facilitates accurate interpretation.

Typically, slice thickness and spacing are equal. For example, if a 10-mm slice thickness is used, the table is incremented 10 mm after each slice. In this way, all areas of the anatomy within the scanning range are covered. Scan protocols in which the slice thickness and spacing are equal are known as **contiguous.** Scans are not always taken in a contiguous fashion, however. In some cases, spacing is less than slice thickness. This practice results in overlapping images. Images may be overlapped if more slices are desired in a small area, such as the vertebral disk space. An overlapping technique also improves multiplanar and three-dimensional reformations. However, taking overlapping slices increases patient radiation exposure. In some cases, spacing is greater than slice thickness, and small areas between slices are not being scanned. For example, if an 8-mm slice thickness is selected with a corresponding 10-mm table increment, a 2-mm section of anatomy is missed between each slice. This technique is used when a large area must be covered and the

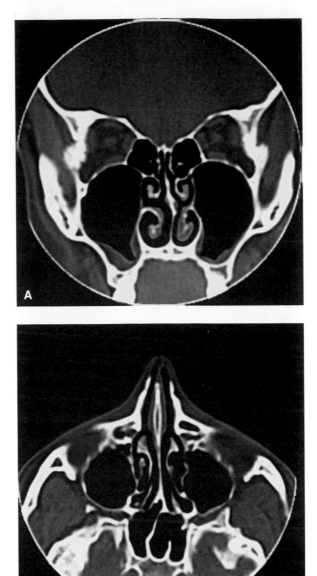

Figure 8–5. *(A)* A sinus slice taken in the coronal plane. *(B)* A sinus slice taken in the axial plane.

suspected lesion is not likely to be small. This technique produces a lower radiation dose to the patient.

PATIENT HISTORY

A history should be taken for all patients. For examinations that require contrast enhancement, the history must include allergies as well as any renal complications. If the patient's chart is accessible, it is helpful to check laboratory reports for the most recent blood urea nitrogen and creatinine values. The normal range varies slightly from facility to facility, but in general, when the blood urea nitrogen value is greater than 30 mg/dl or the creatinine value is greater than 2 mg/dl, a radiologist should be consulted before intravenous contrast medium is administered.

It is important to include in the patient's history any previous medical conditions and surgeries as well as current symptoms. It is also helpful to record when the symptoms began and whether the condition is new or chronic. Because scarring caused by radiation therapy often mimics lung disease, it is important to note previous oncology treatments. Appendix B shows a standard history form used in a CT department.

The practice of obtaining written consent from the patient for the administration of intravenous contrast material is common in some facilities. Acquiring a signed consent form documents that the procedure and risks were discussed with the patient. The practice is not universally accepted. Opponents believe that the process of reading and signing a consent form often increases patient anxiety and increases the likelihood of an adverse reaction. Further, they believe that the forms offer little protection in cases of litigation.

FILMING TECHNIQUES

Filming is the process of copying the image from the cathode-ray tube (CRT) monitor onto sheets of radiographic film. The record produced by this process is referred to as the **hard copy.** Single-emulsion film is used in the CT department. Different formats may be selected that affect the size of the image. Thus, one 11- × 14-inch sheet of film can be used to display different numbers of images. The most popular format for routine filming is 12 images to each sheet of film (called 12 on 1).

The placement of images on the sheet of film varies between institutions. In general, images are placed from left to right in order of location (cephalad to caudad for body scans, caudad to cephalad for head scans).

Controversy arises in studies in which it is necessary to record the same image with more than one window setting, such as the spine. Some radiologists prefer each sheet to contain images filmed at the same window setting, whereas others prefer alternate window settings for each image on the sheet. Another common preference is for the alternate window level images to be placed above and below each other (see Figure 8-6).

For the most part, filming practice is a matter of individual preference and thus can be modified if the situation dictates. When an upgraded camera is purchased, it may be prudent to adjust filming practices to maximize throughput. All CT department staff must allow time to become accustomed to the appearance of the resulting studies.

ARCHIVING METHODS

The process of saving image data from the system disk to an electronic medium is called **archiving.** These archived images can later be retrieved and displayed on the CRT monitor, and refilmed if necessary. More information is available from an image displayed on the monitor than from an image filmed on hard copy and displayed on a view box. Subsequently, most institutions archive image data. Some facilities save data indefinitely, whereas others keep information only for a predetermined period. Because the amount of raw data produced daily is enormous and would require a vast amount of space to save, only the image data are saved.

Several devices are available for archiving. One of the oldest options is magnetic tape, which stores data on large reels. Because this method is slow compared with newer methods, it is rapidly becoming obsolete.

Another option for data storage is the use of 5.25-inch (floppy) or 3.5-inch disks. Because of their limited storage capacity compared with other archiving methods, they are also becoming obsolete.

The newest, most efficient device for storing data is the optical disk. These disks can save approximately 100 times the data saved on the older floppy disks. Two types of optical disks are available. Write once, read many **(WORM)** disks cannot be erased, so data are saved indefinitely. Rewritable magnetic optical disks can be erased so that they can be used repeatedly. The images on both types of optical disk display optimal levels of resolution.

Another new archiving method is digital audiotape (DAT). These tapes resemble standard stereo cassette tapes. Their image resolution is good and is comparable to that of optical disks. They also can be erased and reused. Because the tape must be rewound to the appropriate location, retrieval of data is somewhat slower with DAT tapes compared with optical disks. Individual DAT tapes are less expensive to purchase than optical disks.

CHAPTER SUMMARY

Imaging can be acquired in different planes by adjusting the patient's position. In addition

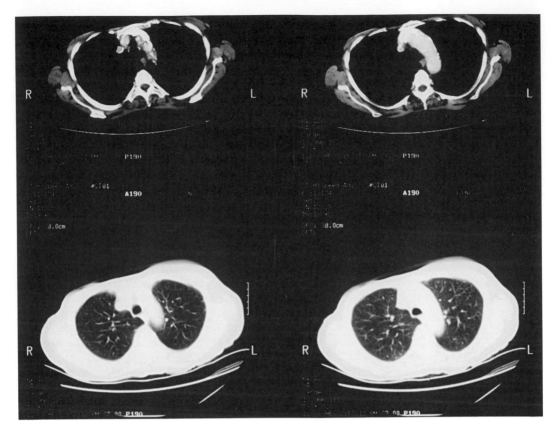

Figure 8–6. The way that images are placed on the film varies greatly among facilities. Camera capabilities and patient throughput should be considered when setting protocols.

to this technique, data can be manipulated retrospectively so that images are created in different planes. Changing patient position to scan in a different plane is done either to better visualize anatomy or to avoid artifacts.

A scout image is obtained to plan the location of the cross-sectional slices. It is essential to input directional information properly so that the scan is correctly annotated as to right–left and anterior–superior orientation. Images should indicate whether contrast material is used.

Clear breathing instructions are necessary for all patients undergoing a body procedure.

It is customary to include in a study a scout image that is cross-referenced. It is also common to include a text screen that includes patient information.

If scans are performed both with and without contrast enhancement, the operator should verify that slices are taken at identical table positions. This practice facilitates comparisons between unenhanced and enhanced images.

Scans are most commonly done in a contiguous fashion. Occasionally, protocols call for overlapping or gapped slices. Changing from contiguous slices to an overlapping or gapped protocol affects the patient radiation exposure.

An appropriate history should be taken for all patients undergoing CT studies. If laboratory values that reflect renal function are available, they should be checked. A radiologist should be notified if any questions arise. A written consent form for contrast administration may or may not be of value, depending on the view of the institution.

A great variation exists in the process of transferring images from the monitor to hard copy. Filming protocols must be adjusted according to specific equipment to maximize patient throughput.

Archiving is the process of saving data on a storage device. Newer systems use optical disks or DAT. Older systems traditionally use magnetic tapes or floppy disks.

REVIEW QUESTIONS

1. Explain how the following planes divide the body: coronal, axial, and sagittal.
2. Which two methods are available to change the plane of an image?
3. In what two situations is it helpful to adjust the image plane?
4. What is the purpose of a scout image?
5. Define contiguous.
6. Why might a scan protocol call for overlapping images?
7. What are the advantages and disadvantages of obtaining consent for contrast medium administration?
8. What does the term WORM refer to on an optical disk?
9. Compared with magnetic tape, floppy disks, and optical disks, what advantage does DAT offer for data storage?

Section II

EXAMINATION PROTOCOLS

Section II discusses specific scanning protocols used to perform standard CT examinations. These protocols should be considered general guidelines. They are not the only accepted methods of scanning; each facility and each radiologist has scanning preferences. Listed in the tables are routine protocols. In some cases, variations are given after the outlined protocol to show a few of the many possible modifications. It is important to remember that hundreds of methods are currently in use. Like all fields of medicine, CT is constantly evolving, with new routines continually being developed. The following chapters explain the rationale behind many common practices.

To optimize the detection of pathologic tissue with CT scanning, the examination must be tailored to each patient.

As was explained in the discussion of contrast enhancement techniques (see Chapter 7), the method of contrast administration in CT continues to be the most controversial and variable aspect of scanning. In addition to the controversy regarding contrast administration among radiologists, techniques vary dramatically according to the type and speed of

the specific scanner. For this reason, suggested techniques for contrast enhancement are given with a broad range of values. Individual CT departments should consider all of the variables in relation to their specific applications when selecting injection techniques.

The protocols outlined are intended for CT examinations in adults. They are written for use with approximately 60% solution of iodinated contrast media containing approximately 280 to 320 mg iodine per milliliter. In general, a biphasic injection technique is used for slow- to moderate-speed scanners. This technique allows an initial bolus to reach peak enhancement; then a slower second phase maintains enhancement throughout the scanning process. Departments with faster scanners, including spiral, or helical, scanners, often use a single bolus injection with a higher flow rate because all scans can be acquired at peak enhancement.

Low-osmolality contrast agents are favored because of their advantages over high-osmolality agents, but the protocols may be used with either. Operators should consult the specific brand of contrast material being used to determine the iodine concentration.

Chapter 9

HEAD AND BRAIN

In scanning the brain, it is important to administer the entire dose of contrast material before scanning begins because the enhancement of most brain lesions results from disruption of the blood-brain barrier, and not from vascularity of the lesion. In most cases, no delay is required between the completion of contrast administration and scanning. A possible exception to this rule is the patient with suspected brain metastasis. Increasing the intravenous contrast dose (200 ml of 60% iodinated contrast media) and waiting approximately 45 minutes after injection may provide better visualization of brain metastasis. Since the advent of magnetic resonance imaging (MRI) in brain cancer staging, this routine, often referred to as **double dose delay,** is much less common.

Scanning is performed after the entire dose of iodinated contrast material is delivered, so exact flow rates are not crucial. For this reason, suggested flow rates are not included in the brain and head protocols. Table 9-1 and Figure 9-1 show the protocol for routine brain scanning.

Imaging the posterior fossa of the brain is a challenge in CT scanning (see Table 9-2). Because of the great difference in beam attenuation ability between the dense bone of the skull and the much less dense tissue of the brain, streak artifacts are common. This inherent limitation may be managed by decreasing slice thickness when scanning the posterior fossa and increasing the kilovolt-peak (kVp) setting.

Ideally, when scanning the pituitary, the coronal and axial planes should be as nearly perpendicular to each other as possible (see

Table 9-1. Routine Brain Scanning Protocol

Scout image	Lateral
Landmark*	Orbital meatal line: angle gantry so slices are parallel with this line
Slice plane	Axial
Intravenous contrast†	Without contrast for new cerebrovascular accidents, new subdural hematoma (less than 1 week), hydrocephalus, cerebral trauma, dementia, suspected atrophy, multiple sclerosis with cerebral signs
	Without contrast, followed by administration of 100–140 ml for exclusion of tumor (including metastasis), arteriovenous malformation, abscess, aneurysm, edema, or cerebritis; for diagnosis of headache, seizure, or old or chronic subdural hematoma
Oral contrast	None
Breath hold	None
Slice thickness‡	5 mm from foramen magnum to petrous ridge
	8–10 mm to vertex
Slice interval	Contiguous
Start location	Foramen magnum
End location	Vertex
Filming	Soft tissue window
	Posterior fossa: 170/40
	Above: 100/30
	Bone window on trauma or postoperative patients: 2500/400

* An alternative landmark is the acanthomeatal line. By adjusting the angle of slices parallel to the acanthomeatal line (rather than the orbital meatal line), the radiation dose to the lens of the eye is reduced.
† Some facilities scan the brain with contrast only rather than both without and with contrast. Contrast dose and delay may be adapted for patients with metastatic disease.
‡ Often a consistent slice thickness of 7 to 10 mm is used throughout the brain.

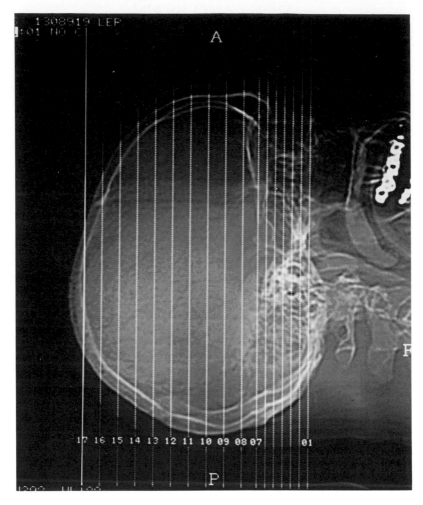

Figure 9–1.   Typical brain protocol. Slices through the posterior fossa are taken at 5-mm thickness, with 10-mm slice thickness used superiorly.

Table 9–2.   Posterior Fossa and Skull Base Screening Protocol

Scout image	Lateral
Landmark*	Orbital meatal line: angle gantry so slices are as nearly perpendicular as possible to this line
Slice plane	Axial, coronal, or both
Intravenous contrast	100–140 ml
Oral contrast	None
Breath hold	None
Slice thickness	3–5 mm
Slice interval	Contiguous
Start location	Axial: suprasellar; coronal: clivus
End location	Axial: hard palate; coronal: anterior orbit
Filming	Soft tissue window: 160/40
	Bone window: 2500/400

* This approach is often referred to as reverse angle image and is designed to reduce beam-hardening artifacts in the posterior fossa and thereby facilitate diagnosis of posterior fossa abnormalities.

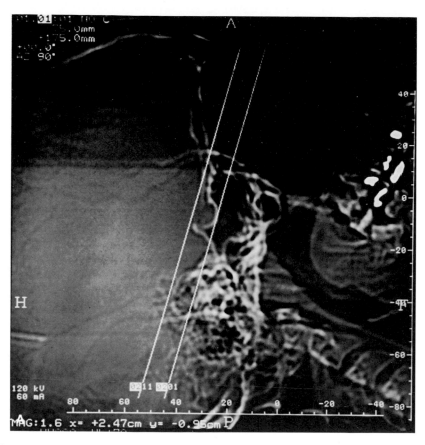

Figure 9–2. *(A)* The lines show the first and last slices in a coronal pituitary study.

Table 9–3. Pituitary and Sella Turcica Screening Protocol

Scout image	Lateral
Landmark	Orbital meatal line: angle gantry so slices are parallel to this line for axial images and perpendicular to it for coronal images; try to avoid dental fillings
Slice plane	Coronal and axial
Intravenous contrast*	100–140 ml
Oral contrast	None
Breath hold	None
Slice thickness	1–1.5 mm
Slice interval	Contiguous
Start location	Coronal: anterior clinoid; axial: just below sellar floor
End location	Coronal: through dorsum; axial: through dorsum sellae
Filming	Soft tissue window: 180/40
	Bone window on images that are reconstructed in a bone algorithm: 2500/400

* Research suggests that scanning after a bolus of intravenous contrast material (at least 2 ml/sec) improves visualization of small pituitary lesions. Some radiologists perfer to perform scans both without and with contrast enhancement.

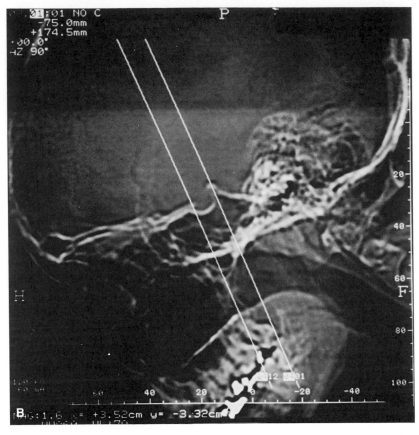

Figure 9–2. *(Continued) (B)* The lines show the first and last slices in an axial pituitary study.

Table 9–4. Internal Auditory Canal Scanning Protocol

Scout image	Lateral
Landmark	Orbital meatal line: angle gantry so slices are parallel with this line for axial images and perpendicular to it for coronal images
Slice plane	Axial, coronal, or both
Intravenous contrast*	Without contrast for temporal bone, petrous bone, hearing loss, cholesteatoma, facial or seventh nerve palsy, mastoiditis, labyrinthitis, or chronic otitis media
	Without contrast, followed by administration of 100–140 ml for acoustic neuroma or sensorineural hearing loss
Oral contrast	None
Breath hold	None
Slice thickness†	3 mm through posterior fossa, 1 mm through canal, 3 mm through petrous bone
Slice interval	Contiguous
Start location	Axial: foramen magnum; coronal: posterior semicircular canal
End location	Axial: through petrous ridge; coronal: anterior margin of the attic
Filming	Soft tissue window: 220/50
	Bone window on images that are reconstructed in a bone algorithm: 2800/600

Note: Magnetic resonance imaging is the preferred study, particularly for the evaluation of acoustic neuroma.
* Some facilities perform the examination with contrast enhancement only (omitting the study without contrast enhancement).
† Slice thickness of 1.5 to 2 mm throughout.

Table 9–5. Orbit and Facial Bone Scanning Protocol

Scout image	Lateral
Landmark	Orbital meatal line: angle gantry so slices are parallel to this line for axial images and perpendicular to it for coronal images
Slice plane	Coronal, axial, or both
Intravenous contrast	Without contrast for blunt trauma, foreign body, or Graves' disease
	100–140 ml for suspected mass or visual disturbance
Oral contrast	None
Breath hold	None
Slice thickness	2–3 mm
Slice interval	Contiguous
Start location	Axial: top of maxillary sinus; coronal: sphenoid sinus
End location	Axial: upper orbital rim; coronal: anterior globe
Filming	Soft tissue window: 150/40
	Bone window on images that are reconstructed in a bone algorithm: 2500/400

Note: To reduce ocular motion, ask the patient to fix his eyes on an object. Three-dimensional reformations may be helpful in cases of orbital fracture. For facial bones, the protocol remains basically unchanged except that the area scanned is enlarged to encompass all facial bones.

Table 9–6. Paranasal Sinus Scanning Protocol

Scout image	Lateral
Landmark	Orbital meatal line: angle gantry so slices are parallel to this line for axial images and perpendicular to it for coronal images
Slice plane	Coronal
Intravenous contrast	Without contrast for sinusitis
	100–140 ml for suspected mass
Oral contrast	None
Breath hold	None
Slice thickness	5 mm through sphenoid, 2–3 mm at ethmoid
Slice interval	Contiguous
Start location	Coronal: dorsum sellae
End location	Coronal: through anterior frontal sinus
Filming	Soft tissue window: 200/40
	Bone window on images: 1600/400

Table 9–7. Temporomandibular Joint Scanning Protocol

Scout image	Lateral
Landmark	Orbital meatal line: angle gantry so slices are parallel to this line for axial images and perpendicular to it for coronal images
Slice plane	Coronal
Intravenous contrast	None
Oral contrast	None
Breath hold	None
Slice thickness	1–3 mm
Slice interval	Contiguous
Start location	Just posterior to joint
End location	Through entire joint
Filming	Soft tissue window: 180/40
	Bone window on images: 2500/400

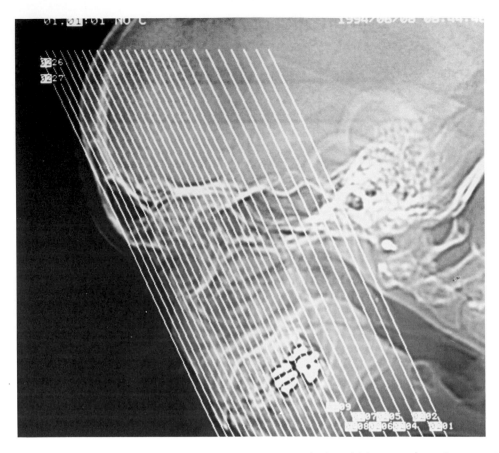

Figure 9–3. The lines show a typical sinus scanning protocol. Slice thickness and spacing are set at 5 mm through the sphenoid sinus and are then decreased to 3 mm at the ethmoid sinus.

Table 9-3). However, if the patient has dental fillings, it is preferable to adjust the angle to avoid as much of the dental filling as possible.

Although the pituitary gland is most often scanned in both the axial and coronal planes, use of the latter plane provides more useful information. Streak artifact from the dense bone of the sella turcica is common in the axial plane and is reduced or eliminated in the coronal plane (see Figure 9-2).

Tables 9-4 through 9-7 and Figure 9-3 show the scanning protocols for the remaining structures of the head.

Chapter 10

NECK

Routine scanning of the neck is typically performed with the patient supine and the neck slightly extended (see Tables 10-1, 10-2). To reduce artifacts that degrade images in the lower neck, the patient should be instructed to lower the shoulders as much as possible. It is not necessary for the patient to hyperextend the neck. Hyperextension of the neck should be avoided in patients with large supraglottic tumors because it may increase the obstruction of the patient's airway.

Often, scans are acquired while the patient performs a modified Valsalva's maneuver (see Table 10-3). This maneuver requires the patient to blow the cheeks out. This technique helps to distend the pyriform sinuses. Another technique used to evaluate the aryepiglottic folds and pyriform sinuses is to ask the patient to pronounce a prolonged ''e'' during scanning.

Table 10–1. Routine Neck Scanning Protocol*

Scout image	Lateral
Landmark	Orbital meatal line
Slice plane	Axial
Intravenous contrast	100–150 ml
	Rate: 1 ml/sec; start scanning after 60 seconds
Oral contrast	None
Breath hold	Quiet respiration
Slice thickness	5 mm
Slice interval	Contiguous
Start location	Just superior to base of tongue
End location	Lung apices
Reconstruction algorithm	Standard or soft
Filming	Soft tissue window: 250/30

* For routine neck or oral pharynx survey to exclude neck mass, parotid gland mass, parathyroid adenoma, or enlarged nodes.

Table 10–2. Neck and Larynx Scanning Protocol

Scout image	Lateral
Landmark	Orbital meatal line
Slice plane	Axial: position patient with neck mildly hyperextended
Intravenous contrast	100 ml
	Rate: 1 ml/sec; start scanning after 60 seconds
Oral contrast	None
Breath hold	Quiet respiration
Slice thickness	3–5 mm
Slice interval	Contiguous
Start location	Just superior to base of tongue
End location	Cricoid cartilage
Reconstruction algorithm	Standard
Filming	Soft tissue window: 250/30

Table 10–3.   Brachial Plexus Scanning Protocol

Scout image	Anteroposterior: include neck and upper chest (patient's arms down)
Landmark	Orbital meatal line
Slice plane	Axial
Intravenous contrast*	80–120 ml
	Rate: 1 ml/sec; start scanning after 60 seconds
Oral contrast	None
Breath hold	Suspended inspiration
Slice thickness	5 mm
Slice interval	Contiguous
Start location	C4
End location	T4
Reconstruction algorithm	Standard
Filming†	Soft tissue window: 330/40
	Scans containing lung also filmed in lung window: 1800/−600

* Because of artifact from dense contrast material, it is best to inject in the arm that is opposite the side of primary interest.
† Some radiologists prefer to review images in a bone window to exclude tumor.

Chapter 11

CHEST

To decrease artifacts created by cardiac motion, the shortest scan time possible should be used in imaging the chest (see Table 11-1). Depending on the type of scanner, short scan times may permit clustering of scans (see Chapter 4). This method can reduce misregistration caused by uneven patient breathing. Spiral scans should be of the longest duration possible. These scans are often limited by tube heating and the length of time the patient can suspend respiration (see Figure 11-1).

The thorax has the highest intrinsic natural contrast of any body part. The pulmonary vessels and ribs have significantly different densities from the adjacent aerated lung. In most adults, the mediastinal vessels and lymph nodes are surrounded by enough fat to be easily identified. Therefore, in most patients, if normal anatomy is known in detail and sequential scans are analyzed carefully, the routine use of intravenous contrast material is unnecessary. However, in some patients, intravenous administration of contrast material may be necessary. The use of intravenous contrast agents should be reserved for a few specific cases: the presence of insufficient mediastinal fat, which makes identification of normal vascular structures difficult; confusion concerning differentiation of a normal variant or congenital anomaly involving a mediastinal vessel from a pathologic process, either a vascular abnormality (e.g., aneurysm) or a soft tissue mass; or the

Table 11–1. Routine Chest Scanning Protocol*

Scout image	Anteroposterior
Landmark	Sternal notch
Slice plane	Axial or spiral
Intravenous contrast†	80–150 ml
	Rate: 1.5–2 ml/sec for 15 seconds, followed by 1 ml/sec; start scanning after 60 seconds
Oral contrast	None
Breath hold	Suspended inspiration
Slice thickness	8–10 mm through apices
	5 mm through hilum (begin thinner section just superior to carina, and continue until through hilum)
	8–10 mm through base of lung
Slice interval	Contiguous
Start location	Sternal notch
End location‡	Through lung bases
Reconstruction algorithm	Standard or detail
Filming	Soft tissue (mediastinal) window: 320/20
	Lung window: 1400/−600

* To exclude or follow up tumor, metastatic disease, or lymphoma.
† Radiologists disagree as to the importance of intravenous contrast enhancement for routine chest studies. Many experts believe that contrast is not necessary under ordinary circumstances and should be used only in specific instances.
‡ Because lung cancer may metastasize to the adrenal glands, scanning is often continued through the adrenals in patients with a history of cancer.

Table 11–2. Chest Scanning Protocol*

Scout image	Anteroposterior
Landmark	Sternal notch
Slice plane	Axial or spiral
Intravenous contrast†	100–150 ml
	Rate: 1.5–2 ml/sec for 15 seconds, followed by 1 ml/sec; start scanning after 25 seconds
Oral contrast	None
Breath hold	Suspended inspiration
Slice thickness	8–10 mm
Slice interval	Contiguous
Start location	Sternal notch
End location	Through lung bases
Reconstruction algorithm	Standard or detail
Filming	Soft tissue (mediastinal) window: 330/30
	Lung window: 1800/−600

* For aortic dissection.
† This protocol is dependent on the use of a fast scanner. Older, slower scanners may necessitate the following revision: Without contrast material, scan through the thoracic aorta for localization. With a bolus of 30–50 ml each, scan at the level of the mid-ascending aorta (both ascending aorta and descending aorta will be on one slice) and again at the arch.

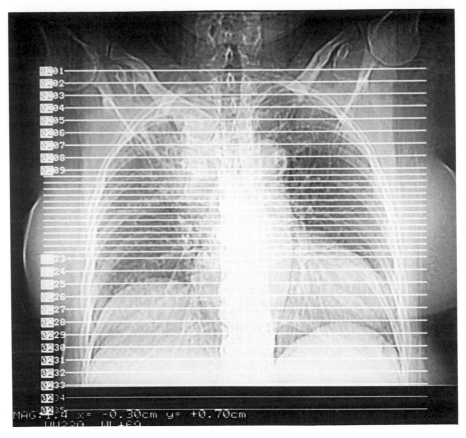

Figure 11–1. Typical chest study. Slices through the hilum are scanned with a thickness and spacing of 5 mm. Slices above and below the hilum are scanned with a thickness and spacing of 10 mm.

Table 11–3. High-Resolution Chest Scanning Protocol*

Scout image	Anteroposterior
Landmark	Sternal notch
Slice plane	Axial
Intravenous contrast	None
Oral contrast	None
Breath hold	Suspended inspiration
Slice thickness	1–1.5 mm
Slice interval	10 mm or at selected levels (aortic arch, hilum, lung bases)
Start location	Sternal notch
End location	Through lung bases
Reconstruction algorithm	Bone
Filming	Lung window: 1800/−600†

* For evaluation of the lung for abnormality such as interstitial disease or subtle air space consolidation.
† Some radiologists prefer each lung to be filmed separately with a small field size so that one lung fills up the screen to further improve image resolution. Additional scans with the patient in a prone position may provide more information.

need for characterization of a lesion by observing its enhancement pattern (e.g., separation of complex pleuroparenchymal abnormality)[1] (see Tables 11–2, 11–3).

REFERENCE

1. Lee J, Sagel S, Stanley R: *Computed Body Tomography with MRI Correlation.* New York, Raven Press, 1989, p 172.

Chapter 12

ABDOMEN

Appropriate contrast enhancement is essential in imaging the abdominal organs, especially the liver. It is important to complete most or all of the study before intravenous contrast medium reaches the equilibrium phase (see Chapter 7). The speed of the scanner is clearly an important factor in reaching this goal.

With older, slower scanners, scanning the entire liver before the equilibrium phase was impossible. Therefore, precontrast scans were acquired to reduce the chance of missing a lesion that becomes isodense at the equilibrium phase of contrast enhancement.

Most scanners available today are much faster. These systems can complete most, if not all, of the study before intravenous contrast material reaches the equilibrium phase. For this reason, many radiologists believe that precontrast scanning is no longer necessary in the abdomen. However, some radiologists continue to use abdominal protocols that include both pre- and postcontrast slices. They believe that although precontrast images are no longer necessary in making a diagnosis of abdominal abnormality, these images help to characterize the lesion. Viewing a suspected abnormality both before and after contrast enhancement may provide significant information about the origin of the lesion.

If precontrast slices are obtained, they are most commonly performed through the liver. Protocols often specify that precontrast images are necessary only in patients with a history of cancer.

If an organ is specified, precontrast slices may be necessary. For example, if an order reads, "Abdomen: attention adrenals, rule out neoplasm," the radiologist probably prefers unenhanced images through the adrenals only, followed by an enhanced study of the entire abdomen. Slice thickness is often adjusted as well.

Precontrast slices are helpful whenever questionable calcifications (e.g., kidney stones) are seen. If only a contrast-enhanced examination is performed, it may be difficult to discern calculi in the iodine-enhanced renal system.

The flow rate of contrast injection is debated within the industry. Rapid injection rates (2 ml/sec or higher) are generally limited to scanners that can perform fast scanning. Even with a high-speed scanning system, the disadvantage of these rapid injection rates must be considered. Rapid injections require placement of a large-bore intravenous catheter (16–18 gauge). Placement of a catheter of this size is often difficult and sometimes impossible. If traditional, high-osmolality contrast medium is used, side effects such as severe flushing or nausea may interrupt scanning.

Another common technique is biphasic injection. This method requires an initial bolus of approximately 50 ml of contrast material at a high injection rate (approximately 2 ml/sec). A slower rate (approximately 0.8 ml/sec) is used until the entire volume is delivered. The bolus phase is used to achieve peak enhancement, whereas the slower second phase is used to extend enhancement time until the scanner completes the study. The increased speed of new scanners permits the use of a single bolus injection at the higher flow rate.

The interval between contrast injection and the beginning of scanning is increasingly critical as scanning speed increases. For example, if a spiral scanning technique is used, data for an entire abdominal study can be obtained in less than 1 minute. This speed allows the operator to determine exactly where he would like to see the contrast. If a delay of 30 seconds after injection is used, it is likely that the contrast material in the liver will be in the arterial phase and will not have reached

Table 12–1. Routine Abdomen
Scanning Protocol

Scout image	Anteroposterior
Landmark	Xiphoid
Slice plane	Axial or spiral
Intravenous contrast	100–120 ml
	Rate: 1.5–2 ml/sec for 15 seconds, followed by 1 ml/sec; start scanning after 60 seconds
Oral contrast	400 ml 45 minutes before scanning and 200 ml just before scanning
Breath hold	Suspended expiration
Slice thickness	8–10 mm
Slice interval	Contiguous
Start location	Lung bases (include all of liver)
End location*	Iliac crest
Reconstruction algorithm	Standard
Filming†	Soft tissue window: 350/50 Lung window (for slices that contain lung): 1600/−600 High-contrast liver window (for slices that contain liver): 150/30

* Terminology differs according to facility. In some institutions, a routine abdomen survey includes the pelvis; therefore, the end location would be the symphysis pubis rather than the iliac crest.
† The high-contrast liver window setting is optional and not routinely used in many facilities.

the venous structures. The kidneys will probably have no contrast enhancement. A 90-second delay will likely show the liver with contrast material in both the arterial and venous structures. The kidneys still may not exhibit significant contrast enhancement.

Because certain metastatic liver lesions are best visualized in the arterial phase, it may be desirable to start scanning after 30 seconds. However, to see contrast enhancement in the renal system, it is necessary to pause scanning when the lower portion of the liver is reached, before the scan reaches the kidney. At a 10-mm table increment, approximately 15 slices are needed. Delaying the scanning process 2 to 3 minutes from the initial injection permits visualization of contrast-enhanced kidneys. If the procedure requires the pelvis to be scanned, scanning must be paused before the bladder is reached. An additional 2- to 3-minute delay increases contrast filling of the bladder.

The use of a short delay (less than 60 seconds) after the initial injection of contrast medium may necessitate repetition of scans

through the liver to permit visualization of the hepatic venous structure. This protocol is used at some medical centers, but it is not widespread. Likely reasons for its limited use include an increase in patient radiation exposure and a decrease in patient throughput.

Determining the best timing for contrast enhancement is largely a matter of personal preference as well as trial and error. Several reports suggest altering injection techniques according to the patient's clinical history, although this approach is not always practical.

The use of oral contrast material is imperative to differentiate a fluid-filled loop of bowel from a mass or an abnormal fluid collection. Either a dilute barium suspension or a dilute water-soluble agent may be used. In general, the greater the volume of oral contrast material, the better the bowel opacification. Although a volume of at least 600 ml is desired, patient compliance may be a limiting factor. Patients should be given only clear liquids for at least 2 hours before scanning to ensure that food in the stomach is not mistaken for pathologic tissue.

Many operators include a region of interest (ROI) measurement of the liver and spleen. A difference of more than 20 Hounsfield units (HU) is an indicator of fatty infiltrate in the liver.

A routine abdomen study is outlined in Table 12-1.

PANCREAS

CT is the imaging method of choice for evaluation of the pancreas.[1] Methods such as ultrasound, plain film radiography, and contrast examination of the gastrointestinal tract may provide additional information, but pancreatic CT provides the most reliable overall data (see Table 12–2).

The pancreas differs in size, shape, and location depending on the individual patient. In general, the pancreas is located between the areas of the twelfth thoracic vertebra (superiorly) and the second lumbar vertebra (inferiorly). A technique that includes the use of thin slices (5 mm or less) and intravenous contrast enhancement improves the likelihood of visualizing the main pancreatic duct. In jaundiced patients, noncontrast scans around the area of the common bile duct may improve visualization of common bile duct calculi. Because the pancreatic head lies in

Table 12–2. Abdomen Scanning Protocol: Attention Pancreas*

Scout image	Anteroposterior
Landmark	Xiphoid
Slice plane	Axial or spiral
Intravenous contrast†	100–150 ml
	Rate: 1.5–2 ml/sec for 15 seconds, followed by 1 ml/sec; start scanning after 60 seconds
Oral contrast	400 ml 30–45 minutes before scanning and 100–200 ml 15 minutes before scanning
Breath hold	Suspended expiration
Slice thickness	8–10 mm from base of lung to top of pancreas (approximately T12–L1)
	5 mm through pancreas (approximately L3)
	8–10 mm to iliac crest
Slice interval	Contiguous
Start location	Lung bases (include all of liver)
End location†	Iliac crest
Reconstruction algorithm	Standard
Filming	Soft tissue window: 350/50
	Lung window (for slices that contain lung): 1600/−600

* For pancreatic cancer, pancreatic pseudocyst, acute pancreatitis, or jaundice.
† Often precontrast slices through the pancreas are performed.

such close proximity to the small bowel, the patient must be given oral contrast material immediately before scanning. Often, it is difficult to differentiate the margins of the pancreas from the duodenum. In such cases, it may be helpful to obtain additional slices with the patient lying in a right decubitus position.

ADRENALS

CT is the primary radiologic imaging method for evaluating the adrenals (see Table 12–3). Most adrenal masses are detected with an 8- to 10-mm (contiguous) slice thickness. If small masses are suspected, a thinner slice is indicated (3–5 mm). The adrenals are usually scanned with contrast enhancement. However, as in most other CT examinations, many protocol variations are used. Many facilities use a few precontrast slices through the adrenals followed by a contrast-enhanced study.

KIDNEYS

Intravenous excretory urography is the major screening test for the detection of renal

Table 12–3. Abdomen Scanning Protocol: Attention Adrenals*

Scout image	Anteroposterior
Landmark	Xiphoid
Slice plane	Axial or spiral
Intravenous contrast†	100–150 ml
	Rate: 1.5–2 ml/sec for 15 seconds followed by 1 ml/sec; start scanning after 60 seconds
Oral contrast	400 ml 30–45 minutes before scanning and 100–200 ml just before scanning
Breath hold	Suspended expiration
Slice thickness	8–10 mm from base of lung to top of adrenals
	3–5 mm through adrenals
	8–10 mm to iliac crest
Slice interval	Contiguous
Start location	Lung bases (include all of liver)
End location	Iliac crest
Reconstruction algorithm	Standard
Filming	Soft tissue window: 350/50
	Lung window (for slices that contain lung): 1600/−600

* For adrenal mass, Cushing's syndrome, aldosteronoma, or pheochromocytoma.
† Intravenous contrast material is not recommended in patients with pheochromocytoma because it may cause a hypertensive crisis. Glucagon is also contraindicated because it is a potent adrenal stimulant. It may be necessary to scan to the level of the symphysis pubis because a small percentage of pheochromocytomas are related to the bladder. Often precontrast slices of the adrenals are performed.

Table 12–4. Abdomen Scanning Protocol: Attention Kidney

Scout image	Anteroposterior
Landmark	Xiphoid
Slice plane	Axial or spiral
Intravenous contrast*	100–150 ml
	Rate: 1.5–2 ml/sec for 15 seconds, followed by 1 ml/sec; start scanning after 60 seconds
Oral contrast	400 ml 30–45 minutes before scanning and 100–200 ml just before scanning
Breath hold	Suspended expiration
Slice thickness†	8–10 mm†
Slice interval	Contiguous
Start location	Lung bases (include all of liver)
End location	Iliac crest
Reconstruction algorithm	Standard
Filming	Soft tissue window: 350/50
	Lung window (for slices that contain lung): 1600/−600

* Precontrast slices through the kidney are occasionally indicated.
† Some radiologists prefer thinner slices (5 mm) through the kidneys.

masses, but CT examination can add significant information to the diagnosis. Although ultrasound is highly accurate in differentiating between a cystic lesion and a solid renal neoplasm, CT is often preferred for staging renal neoplasms because it provides a better topographic display of perirenal spaces[1] (see Table 12-4).

Generally, precontrast images are not helpful unless the presence of renal calculi, perinephric hematoma, or a calcified mass is suspected.

REFERENCE

1. Balfe D, Peterson R, Van Dyke J: Normal abdominal and pelvic anatomy. In *Computed Body Tomography*, 2nd ed. Edited by Lee J, Sagel S, Stanley R. New York, Raven Press, 1989, p 767.

Chapter 13

PELVIS

CT provides an excellent cross-sectional display of bony and soft tissue pelvic structures, regardless of body type. For this reason, it is an important imaging tool for evaluating patients suspected of having pelvic disease (see Table 13-1).

Careful patient preparation is essential in imaging the pelvis. Complete opacification of the many loops of small bowel that are present in the pelvis is necessary so that fluid-filled bowel is not mistaken for a mass or an abnormal fluid collection. Either a dilute barium suspension (1%–2%) or a dilute water-soluble agent (2%–4%) can be used. A minimum of 600 ml of oral contrast material (1000 ml is preferable) should be given 1 to 2 hours before scanning. Although the rectosigmoid colon usually can be distinguished by its location and fecal content, opacification of this anatomy is sometimes required. Opacification of the rectosigmoid colon is often accomplished by giving the patient oral contrast material 6 to 12 hours before scanning. In some cases, 150 ml of a dilute water-soluble agent (1%–3%) is administered by enema. A few institutions use positive contrast by inserting air through a rectal tube. When air is used, pelvic scans are typically obtained with the patient in the prone position.

In women, a tampon can be inserted in the vagina to aid in identification of the vaginal canal.

Most facilities routinely use intravenous contrast material for examinations of the pelvis.

Imaging when the urinary bladder is distended is often helpful because the distended bladder may displace small bowel loops and facilitate identification of other pelvic structures.

Table 13-1. Routine Pelvis Scanning Protocol*

Scout image	Anteroposterior
Landmark	Iliac crest
Slice plane	Axial or spiral
Intravenous contrast	100–120 ml
	Rate: 1–1.5 ml/sec; start scanning 2–3 minutes after all contrast material is delivered
Oral contrast†	600–100 ml 1–2 hours before scanning
Breath hold	Suspended expiration or normal respiration
Slice thickness	8–10 mm
Slice interval‡	Contiguous
Start location	Iliac crest
End location	Symphysis pubis
Reconstruction algorithm	Standard
Filming§	Soft tissue window: 400/20

* For diverticulitis, appendicitis, lower quadrant pain, pelvic inflammatory disease, mass, rectal cancer, or bladder cancer.

† Patient may be given 300 ml dilute barium suspension 6 to 12 hours before scanning to improve the likelihood of opacification of the rectosigmoid colon.

‡ Many facilities use an 8- or 10-mm slice thickness in conjunction with a 10- to 20-mm table increment.

§ Because pelvic malignancies may metastasize to bone, it may be necessary to view or film images in a bone setting as well as a soft tissue setting.

Chapter 14

SPINE

Compared with conventional radiography, CT examinations of the spine produce images with inherently high soft tissue contrast. This contrast permits the visualization of structures such as the intervertebral disks, ligaments, muscles, and vessels, as well as bone detail (see Tables 14–1, 14–2, 14–3). Visualization of intradural structures is improved by the intrathecal administration of water-soluble contrast material. CT examinations are performed after myelography to enhance or clarify myelographic findings of intradural and extradural abnormalities.

Magnetic resonance imaging (MRI) provides even higher soft tissue sensitivity than CT, and in certain circumstances, it is the modality of choice for imaging the spine (e.g., multiple sclerosis, hydromyelia, syringomyelia). For some conditions, such as spinal steno-

Table 14–2. Thoracic Spine Scanning Protocol*

Scout image	Anteroposterior and lateral
Landmark	Sternal notch or xiphoid
Slice plane	Axial: angle gantry so slices will be parallel with most interspaces
Intravenous contrast	None
Oral contrast	None
Breath hold	Inspiration
Slice thickness	5 mm
Slice interval	Contiguous
Start location	Pedicle above area of interest
End location	Pedicle below area of interest
Reconstruction algorithm	Standard or detail
Filming	Soft tissue window: 250/50 Bone window: 1800/400

* For degenerative disk disease, metastatic bone disease, neoplasm, or trauma.

Table 14–1. Routine Cervical Spine Scanning Protocol*

Scout image	Anteroposterior and lateral
Landmark	Orbital meatal line
Slice plane	Axial: angle gantry so slices will be parallel with most interspaces (see Figure 14-1)
Intravenous contrast	None
Oral contrast	None
Breath hold	Quiet respiration
Slice thickness	2–4 mm
Slice interval†	Contiguous
Start location	Pedicle of C3
End location	Through C7
Reconstruction algorithm	Standard or detail
Filming	Soft tissue window: 250/50 Bone window: 1800/400

* For degenerative disk disease, herniated disk, neoplasm, infection, or trauma.
† Often performed with a 1-ml overlap, such as a 2-mm slice interval used with a 3-mm slice thickness. This procedure is used to obtain more slices through the disk space and improve the quality of reformatted images.

sis, MRI is equivalent to CT. In some situations, CT is considered superior to MRI, such as in the evaluation of bony abnormalities of the spine (see Figure 14-1).

It is not practical to perform a CT examination of the entire spinal column as is done in conventional radiography. Because of the many axial slices required, CT is not intended as a general survey examination of the spine. Instead, specific areas (generally limited to three to four disk spaces) should be identified before the start of the CT examination.

Radiologists disagree as to the optimal protocol for scanning the spine, particularly the lumbar spine. There are two common approaches to spine imaging in CT. The first consists of angling the gantry so that all slices are taken directly through the intervertebral spaces (see Figure 14-2). This technique requires the operator to adjust the gantry tilt at each vertebral level examined. This approach may produce the best axial images, but it is impossible to reformat images acquired at

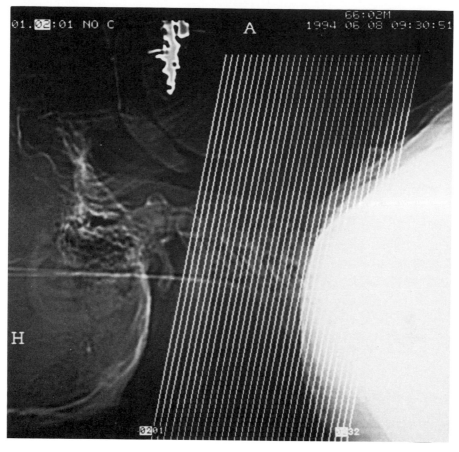

Figure 14–1. The lines represent a typical cervical spine protocol.

Table 14–3. Lumbar Sacral Spine Scanning Protocol*

Scout image	Anteroposterior and lateral
Landmark	Xiphoid or iliac crest
Slice plane	Axial: angle gantry so slices will be parallel with most interspaces (see Figures 14-2 and 14-3)
Intravenous contrast	None
Oral contrast	None
Breath hold	Quiet respiration
Slice thickness	5 mm
Slice interval†	Contiguous
Start location	Pedicle of L3
End location	S1
Reconstruction algorithm	Standard or detail
Filming	Soft tissue window: 250/50
	Bone window: 1800/400

* For degenerative disk disease, herniated disk, neoplasm, or trauma.
† Often performed with a 1-mm overlap; for example, a 4-mm slice interval is used with a 5-mm slice thickness. This procedure is used to obtain more slices through the disk space and improve the quality of reformatted images. Scanning may be done in a semicontiguous fashion, for example, contiguous from pedicle to pedicle, through the first disk space. The gantry angle is then adjusted to match the next disk space, which is scanned pedicle to pedicle, and so on through S1.

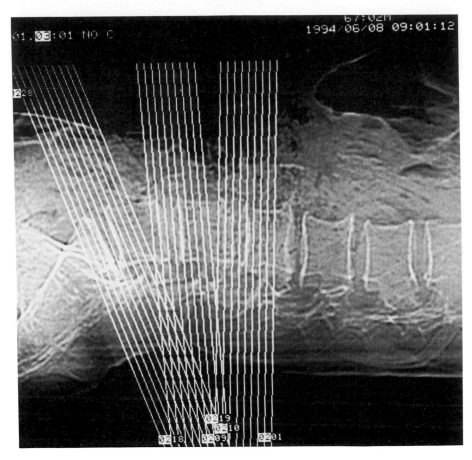

Figure 14–2. Typical lumbar spine protocol that uses a gantry tilt that is adjusted according to each individual disk space.

varying gantry tilts. Some radiologists prefer this technique because they believe that obtaining images in this way prevents the false appearance of a bulging disk. The opposing view is that the appearance of a bulging disk cannot be created, regardless of the image plane. The second protocol requires slices to be taken in a contiguous fashion, with the gantry tilt consistent throughout the study (Figure 14–3). This method allows reformations that include the entire scanned area.

If the second method is used, the images can be reformatted to produce images that mimic scans acquired with a gantry tilt (see Chapter 5).

In general, intravenous contrast medium is not used in CT scanning of the spine. However, some radiologists prefer to use intravenous contrast enhancement for the diagnosis

of degenerative disk disease because the epidural space will become enhanced, making subtle disk herniations clearer. Another common reason for intravenous contrast enhancement is to aid in differentiating disk from surgical scar tissue.

Scans are often obtained after intrathecal contrast material is given for a myelography study. Intrathecal contrast medium may be helpful for the diagnosis of degenerative disk disease and other disk diseases, such as an extradural neoplasm. Most reports suggest a delay of 1 to 4 hours between the intrathecal injection and scanning. This delay allows the contrast material to dilute. If the scans are performed while the contrast material is too dense, intradural structures may be masked. Another technique often used for postmyelography CT scanning is rolling the patient

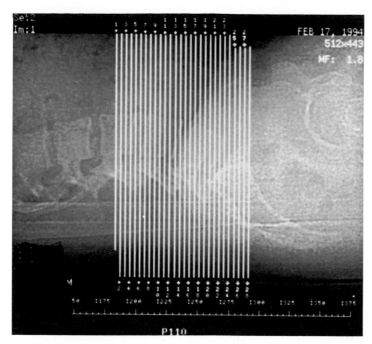

Figure 14–3. Typical lumbar spine study. The cuts are done in a contiguous fashion with a 5-mm slice thickness.

over before transferring her to the CT table. This maneuver prevents the layering of contrast material and cerebrospinal fluid.

Proper localization is essential in scanning the spine. For this reason, it is common to obtain an anteroposterior scout projection in addition to a lateral scout image. Obtaining the anteroposterior view permits vertebral

levels to be more readily counted and classified to ensure that scans are taken at the appropriate levels. When scanning the lumbar spine, it is important to note whether the patient has a sixth lumbar vertebra that requires additional scans. If prior radiographs are available and can be evaluated before scanning, only a lateral scout is necessary.

Chapter 15

MUSCULOSKELETAL SYSTEM

Along with magnetic resonance imaging (MRI), CT is a major method for the evaluation of musculoskeletal anatomy and disease. CT is helpful in providing specific information about bone or other mineralized tissue. It is also a useful method of evaluating bone and soft tissue tumors. It adds details to information obtained with conventional radiography in cases of multiple fractures (e.g., in the pelvis). CT is also used to evaluate joints, especially after air or iodinated contrast material is injected into the joint.

CT of the musculoskeletal system offers several advantages: (1) display of cross-sectional anatomy and spatial relationships, (2) ability to image both sides of the body to permit comparison, (3) ability to display bone and soft tissue components simultaneously, (4) excellent contrast sensitivity, and (5) ability to perform multiplanar and three-dimensional reformation retrospectively.

The techniques used to scan the musculoskeletal system are tailored to each patient (see Table 15-1). Patients should be positioned carefully so that both sides are as symmetric as possible. The lower extremities are usually scanned with the patient supine and placed feet first into the scanner. The upper extremities are scanned with the patient supine and placed head first into the scanner. A scout image is taken to localize the area of interest. Often, it is helpful to obtain a lateral view as well as an anteroposterior projection scout view. In general, the plane of CT section should be perpendicular to the region of interest (ROI).

The patient should be made as comfortable as possible with pillows and angle sponges so that inadvertent motion does not degrade the study. Depending on the area and abnormality in question, there is wide variation in the positioning of the patient. For example, the ankles are usually scanned with the feet flat against the table and the gantry angled. However, this position is often modified so that the patient extends his legs straight out and the gantry is perpendicular to the lower leg.

Slice thickness varies according to the size of the lesion and the area to be scanned. Most soft tissue and bone tumors are visualized with a slice thickness of 8 to 10 mm. If the lesions are small, or if fractures are suspected, it may be necessary to decrease the slice thickness to 3 to 5 mm. If fine detail is required, small areas may be scanned at a slice thickness of 1 to 3 mm. These thin slices may be used to evaluate tibial plateau or wrist fractures. Multiplanar and three-dimensional reformations may be particularly helpful in the evaluation of fractures.

Intravenous contrast medium is not routinely administered, but it may be helpful in specific cases. Intravenous contrast administration may be helpful in evaluating the vascularity of a tumor or in showing the relation of major arteries or veins to musculoskeletal masses.

Table 15-1. Overview of Musculoskeletal Scanning Protocol

Scout image	Anteroposterior (lateral view is helpful in certain situations)
Landmark	Center of region being examined
Slice plane	Axial or spiral
Intravenous contrast	None*
Oral contrast	None
Breath hold	Normal respiration
Slice thickness	Depends on part examined
Slice interval	Contiguous
Start location	2–3 cm above suspected abnormality
End location	2–3 cm below suspected abnormality
Reconstruction algorithm	Standard (additional images may be reconstructed in a bone algorithm)
Filming	Soft tissue window: 400/20 Bone window: 2000/400

* Intravenous contrast may aid in evaluating tumor vascular structures.

Chapter 16

SPECIALIZED CT STUDIES

A number of specialized CT studies are performed in a variety of clinical settings. Some of these specialized examinations (e.g., dental scanning, bone mineral densitometry) require the purchase of additional computer software as well as ancillary hardware. In other instances, special procedures are performed with only the basic scanning hardware.

Because this text is an introduction to the modality, a detailed analysis of each of these special studies is beyond its scope. However, the reader should be acquainted with the basic goals of these procedures.

BONE DENSITOMETRY

The relation of bone density to bone strength is verified by many investigators. Reduced bone density is associated with greater susceptibility to fractures.

CT offers a method for noninvasive measurement of bone density with the purchase of a bone densitometry package. Sometimes these packages are offered by the scanner manufacturer; however, excellent packages are also available from independent firms. These packages are designed to be used with virtually any type of CT scanner.

Quantitative CT bone densitometry is performed with a standard CT scanner and a bone equivalent calibration phantom and analysis software. The patient lies on top of the calibration phantom, which is positioned in a foam pad. The phantom is scanned simultaneously with the patient.

A lateral scout image is taken to provide localization. Slices are prescribed at the midplane of three vertebral bodies. An area of trabecular bone is defined in each CT image acquired. Region of interest (ROI) measurements are located on the phantom samples. Typically, the examination is performed in 10 minutes or less. The software performs an analysis and determines the degree of osteoporosis present in the patient (see Figure 16-1).

DENTAL SCAN

Specialized dental scanning requires the purchase of additional CT software. This software is sometimes offered by the manufacturer of the CT system, but it can also be purchased from independent software vendors and adapted to the scanner. By creating two- and three-dimensional models, the software allows preoperative planning of dental implants, reconstructive surgery, and trauma surgery. Using this software in planning dental implants allows the clinician to determine exactly how each implant affects the patient's anatomy in all three dimensions simultaneously. Dental software may also allow the clinician to evaluate the quality and quantity of available bone when selecting the size and number of root-form implants. Dental packages often allow the clinician to prepare and evaluate several treatment plans and to select the best option for the patient (see Figure 16-2).

Dental scanning includes the following steps:

1. The patient is positioned supine on the CT table. The scan plane is dictated by the software manufacturer.
2. A scan appliance or a tongue depressor wrapped with gauze is placed in the patient's mouth.
3. A lateral scout view is taken.
4. A series of axial slices are programmed according to the area of interest (i.e., maxilla, mandible). A typical maxillary study consists of approximately 30 slices, whereas a study of the mandible usually consists of 40 slices. Slices are taken at narrow collimation (1-1.5 mm) and in a contiguous fashion.
5. The images are reformatted according to the software manufacturer's instructions.

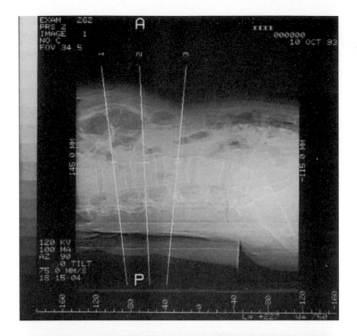

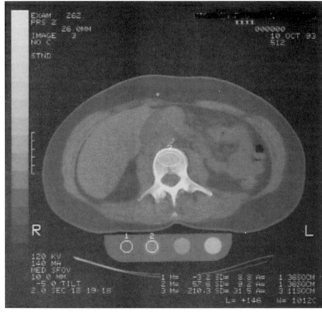

Figure 16–1. Images from a QCT bone mineral densitometry examination. Courtesy of Image Analysis, Inc.

THREE-DIMENSIONAL SPIRAL CT ANGIOGRAPHY

Since the introduction of spiral scanning, researchers have found many new applications for its use. Spiral scanning permits rapid acquisition of image data without an interscan delay, so intravenous contrast material can be imaged entirely during the arterial or venous phase of circulation. This type of data collection provides high-quality three-dimensional angiographic reconstructions.

The procedure for three-dimensional spiral angiography includes the following steps:

1. An intravenous line with an 18-gauge angiography catheter is placed in the antecubital vein.

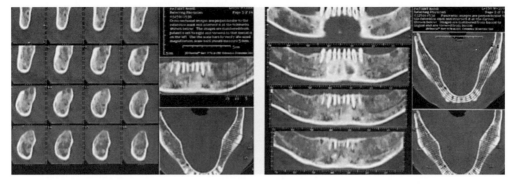

Figure 16–2. Cross-sectional *(left)* and panoramic *(right)* dental scans. Courtesy of Columbia Scientific, Inc.

2. A test injection is performed so that the proper timing can be determined for the contrast bolus to reach the ROI.

3. After the correct delay is determined, a spiral scan is done with a 30-second breath hold. Slice thickness is typically set at 3 mm. Table pitch varies from 1:1 to 2:1. Approximately 125 to 150 ml of low-osmolar iodinated contrast medium is given at a rate of 4 to 5 ml/sec.

4. The data are reconstructed with over-lapping incrementation to provide smoother three-dimensional images.

5. Three-dimensional reformations are produced in one of three reconstruction formats: conventional transaxial image, shaded surface display, or maximum intensity projection.

Although the technique is still in its infancy, clinical data are promising. Because CT angiography is less invasive, less expensive, and

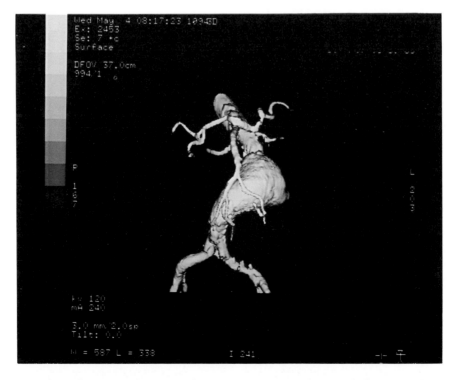

Figure 16–3. Three-dimensional angiography images. Courtesy of General Electric Medical Systems.

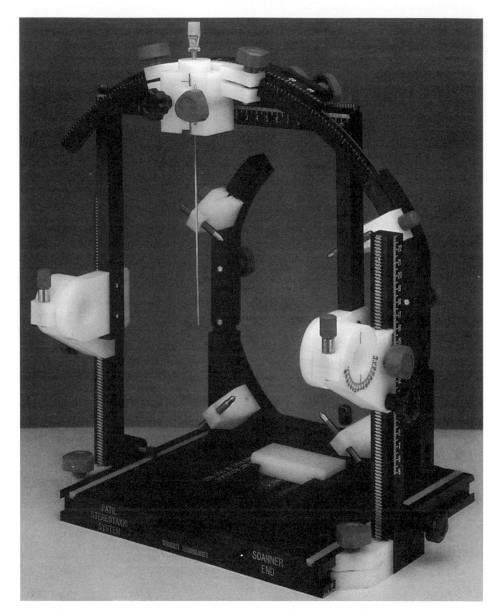

Figure 16–4. Stereotactic system. Courtesy of Westco Medical Corporation.

easier to perform than conventional angiography, it may be an acceptable alternative in some cases (see Figure 16–3).

STEREOTACTIC SURGICAL PLANNING

The use of a stereotactic device in conjunction with CT imaging can provide essential information for the neurosurgeon. This system can provide exact localization of a specific pathologic target.

All stereotactic systems require the purchase of a localizing device. This hardware is placed on the CT scanning table. The patient is positioned so that the head is immobilized within the stereotactic holder. Some systems require the purchase of additional computer software.

Stereotactic systems are used for the following applications:

1. Biopsy of intracranial lesions: brain tumors, inflammatory and parasitic lesions, other unknown lesions

2. Aspiration of cysts
3. Aspiration of brain abscesses and instillation of antibiotics
4. Functional neurosurgery
5. Intracavitary and interstitial irradiation
6. Stereotactic radiosurgery
7. Stereotactic transsphenoidal chemical hypophysectomy
8. Stereotactic laser microsurgery

The procedure for stereotactic planning includes the following steps, although the protocol is dependent on the manufacturer of the stereotactic device:

1. With the patient in the stereotactic head holder, scanning is performed through the area of interest. From these images, the slice that best defines the target is chosen. The scan table is moved to the target plane. Using the localizer light on the CT scanning system, the z coordinate is used to match the specified area on the stereotactic device, and the position is locked on the holder.
2. Using the cursor, the distance from the target to the top of the base platform (y axis) is measured. After the y coordinate

is adjusted according to the manufacturer's instructions, the position is locked.
3. Using the cursor, the lateral distance from the target to the center midline (x axis) is measured. After the x coordinate is adjusted on the stereotactic holder according to the manufacturer's guidelines, the position is locked.

This process sets the coordinate to place the target at the center of the arc. The arc can then be rotated through any desired angle and the target approached at any point on the arc. Therefore, the target can be approached from any point on the skull.

The accuracy of the stereotactic approach depends on the slice thickness of the CT images and the diameter of the scan field. The thinner the slice and the smaller the diameter of scanning, the greater the accuracy. One stereotactic manufacturer reports accuracy up to 0.3 mm for the x and y coordinates and up to 0.6 mm for the z coordinate with a 1.5-mm slice thickness and a scan diameter of 25 cm (see Figure 16–4).[1]

REFERENCE

1. Lunsford LD: *Modern Stereotactic Neurosurgery.* Boston, Martinus Nijhoff, 1988.

Chapter 17

INTERVENTIONAL CT

CT is a valuable tool for use in interventional procedures such as biopsies and abscess drainage. The use of CT to guide percutaneous procedures offers several advantages. High-resolution CT images provide precise three-dimensional localization of lesions. CT images permit the clinician to plan an access route to the lesion by showing the relation of surrounding structures. Because the tip of the needle within the structure can be visualized, procedures can be performed on small lesions. Improving the accuracy of the procedure diminishes the associated risks. Patients can be placed in a variety of positions to allow easier access to the lesion.

CT is most useful in the retroperitoneum (e.g., adrenal glands, lymph nodes, pancreas), pelvis (e.g., lymph nodes), and mediastinum, and for small lesions or collections less than 3 cm in diameter, masses located near major vascular structures, intra-abdominal lesions surrounded by loops of bowel, and lesions that are not easily shown by either ultrasound or fluoroscopy.[1]

In theory, the risk associated with needle biopsy increases as needle diameter increases. When a cutting needle is used, the risk is even greater. However, the overall complication rate is small, approximately 2%.[1] The primary complication of biopsy procedures is bleeding. Highly vascularized lesions increase this risk. A bleeding disorder is a contraindication to percutaneous biopsy. However, patients are often treated with blood products or medications to temporarily remedy the disorder so that the biopsy can be performed.

Biopsy can be performed on virtually any scanner without the purchase of additional computer software, but some supplies, such as specialized needles, are required (see Table 17-1).

The purpose of CT-guided biopsy is to document neoplastic disease (primary, metastatic, or recurrent) or to differentiate neoplastic disease from other processes, such as inflammatory disease, postoperative changes, post-therapeutic changes, or normal structures.

Therefore, the goal in a biopsy procedure is to obtain an adequate sample for laboratory evaluation with minimal trauma to surrounding tissues. This goal is achieved with accurate and expedient placement of the needle.

CT-guided biopsy is not a complicated procedure. It can be broken down into several basic steps.

1. The procedure is explained to the patient and written consent is obtained.
2. Appropriate laboratory values are obtained. Most laboratory evaluations include prothrombin time, partial thromboplastin time, and platelet count.
3. The scan is plotted. This process includes careful review of the patient's previous CT study to determine the optimal patient position, whether oral or intravenous contrast medium is indicated, and the appropriate level for the biopsy.
4. The scan is performed through the selected area. An important consideration in scanning for a biopsy procedure is patient breathing. Clear instructions are essential so that each breath is as similar as possible. The breathing command should be given for each slice (or group of slices, if cluster or spiral scanning is possible). As the needle is placed, the patient is again asked to suspend breathing.
5. The best location for needle entry is selected, and a metallic marker is placed on the skin with the localizer light on the CT scanner.
6. The scan is repeated to confirm the suitability of the selected entry location.
7. With the distance measurement on the CT system, the distance from the

Table 17–1. Supplies for Biopsy and Drainage Procedures

Personal protective equipment*
  Face shields
  Sterile gowns
  Sterile gloves
  Foot covering
Sterile 4 × 4 gauze sponges
Sterile drape
Sterile needles (18, 21, 23 gauge)
Sterile syringes
Scalpel
Needles
  Spinal needles (18, 20, 22 gauge)
  Chiba (20, 22 gauge; 15, 20 cm)
  Trucut and Lee (14, 16, 18 gauge)
  Franseen (18, 20 gauge)
Automatic Gore Biopsy System (biopsy gun)
  20 gauge/15 cm
  18 gauge/16 cm
  22 gauge/15 cm
  20 gauge/16 cm
  20 gauge/20 cm
Metallic skin markers
Skin marking pen
Betadine
1% lidocaine
Catheters
  Pigtail catheter (8, 10 French)
  Sump catheter (12, 14 French)
Fascial dilators (6, 8, 10 French)
Guide wires (0.025 m, 0.038 J-tipped)
Tubes for laboratory studies
Aerobic and anaerobic culture tubes
Formalin or nonbacteriostatic saline
Albuminized glass slides
Suture (nylon or Prolene)
Drainage bag and connecting tubing

---

* Personal protective equipment is mandated by the Occupational Health and Safety Administration (OSHA), Federal Register 1910.1030, Blood Borne Pathogen Standard, effective December 1991.

marker on the patient's skin to the lesion is measured. This measure determines the optimal depth and angle for needle placement.

8. The patient's skin is prepared according to aseptic procedure guidelines. A sterile drape is applied, a local anesthetic (lidocaine 1%) is administered, and the biopsy needle is placed.

9. The scan is repeated (5-mm slice thickness is typical) at the needle location as well as one slice above and one slice below the expected needle location until the tip of the needle is visualized.

10. If the CT image confirms the correct location of the needle, a tissue sample is taken and prepared according to laboratory protocols.

11. Postprocedure scans are taken at 10-mm slice thickness to identify complications such as pneumothorax or hematoma.

The features that make CT an excellent choice for guiding a needle biopsy are also beneficial in performing percutaneous abscess drainage.

Fluid collections that respond the most favorably to percutaneous abscess drainage are well defined, unilocular, free-flowing, and accessible. Often, abscess drainage is performed under less favorable conditions (e.g., fluid collection is multiloculated, composed of necrotic tissue, or poorly defined) if the patient is a poor surgical candidate.

The needle placement technique duplicates that used in percutaneous biopsy. In general, the shortest, straightest access route to the collection is favored. However, care should be taken to avoid major vessels, bowel loops, and the pleural space. After the needle is placed, a drainage catheter is situated. After the catheter is in place, the collection is aspirated as completely as possible. Catheters are usually left to gravity drainage. When drainage is complete, the catheter is withdrawn gradually.

REFERENCE

1. Picus D, Weyman PJ, Anderson DJ: Interventional computed tomography. In *Computed Body Tomography*. New York, Raven Press, 1989, p 94.

Appendix A: Terminology Comparison Chart

Definition of Function	Manufacturer							
	General Electric	Siemens	Picker	Toshiba	Technicare	Philips	Shimadzu	Elscint
Anteroposterior, lateral, etc., digital x-ray image	Scout	Topogram	Pilot	Scanogram/ scanoscope	Delta view/ DVI	Scanogram	CR image	Surview
Display field size	DFOV	Target/zoom	Image size	FOV	Zoom	DFOV	Zoom/ area	FOV
Resolution	Algorithm	Algorithm	Algorithm	FC numbers	Convulver filters	Convolution filters	CR filter	Filter
Space between axials	Increment	Table feed	Couch increment	Interval	Increment	Index	Step	Increment
Continuous scanning	Helical	Spiral	Spiral	Helical	N/A	Volume	N/A	Spiral
Reprocessing raw data to create a new image	Retrospective reconstruction	Review	Reprocessing	Recon reprocessing	REC	Recon zoom	Real-time zoom	Reconstruction
Changing reconstruction priority	Priority reconstruction	Instant image	N/A	Urgent	N/A	Priority recon	Priority recon	Sort
Indicating axial location on digital x-ray image	Cross-reference	Topogram evaluation	Pilot acquisition plan	Slice position display scano CT	SSP	Slice line display	Slice plan	Posted surview
Using image data to create other planes	Reformation	MPR	Reformation	MPR	Reconstruction	MP reformat	Arbitrary angle reformat	Oblique reformat
Image capacity on system disk	Image space	Disk space	Disk space	Image space	Disk space	File space	Disk space	Disk space

N/A = feature not available.

Appendix B: Computed Tomography Patient Medical History

Name _____   File no. _____

Age _____   Sex _____   OP/ER/IN   Date _____

Region examined _____ without/with   Referring data: _____

Region examined _____ without/with   _____

Pertinent clinical data _____

Head		
Headaches	No	Yes
Weakness	No	Yes
Dizziness	No	Yes
Seizures	No	Yes

When did symptoms begin? _____

Surgical history _____

Asthma	No	Yes	Heart disease		No	Yes		
Hypertension	No	Yes	Diabetes		No	Yes	NIDDM	IDDM
Pregnancy	No	Yes	Renal disease		No	Yes	BUN _____	Creatinine _____
Cancer	No	Yes	Type _____					
			Chemo	No Yes	Rad. Tx	No Yes	When? _____	

Pertinent radiology exams _____

Ever had iodine before?   No   Yes   Unsure   **Previous CT scan?** No   Yes   **IVU?** No   Yes

Previous reaction to iodine?   No   Yes   Describe _____

ALLERGIES   NKA   Yes _____

Type of contrast administered: Ionic   Nonionic

Adverse reaction _____

Medication administered _____

R.T. Comments _____

_____ History taken by (Tech/Nurse) _____

99

Glossary

air-contrast interface artifact—Streak artifact caused by a significant difference in density between contrast and air.

aliasing effect—Artifacts that appear on the CT image as fine lines. They occur when too few samples are acquired. Also called sampling artifacts.

archiving—Saving data on auxiliary devices, such as optical disk or digital audiotape, for the purpose of reviewing at a later date.

artifact—Manifestation that is seen on the image but is not present in the object scanned.

attenuation profile—Result of the CT process that accounts for the attenuation properties of each ray sum relative to the position of the ray.

axial plane—Imaginary plane that divides the body into upper and lower sections.

back projection—Process of converting the data from the attenuation profile to a matrix.

beam attenuation—Phenomenon by which an x-ray beam passing through a structure is decreased in intensity or amount because of absorption and interaction with matter. The alteration in the beam varies with the density of the structure it passes through.

beam hardening artifact—Artifacts that result from lower-energy photons being preferentially absorbed, leaving higher-intensity photons to strike the detector array.

bolus phase—Phase of contrast enhancement that immediately follows an intravenous bolus injection. Characterized by an attenuation difference of 30 or more Hounsfield units between the aorta and the inferior vena cava.

bow tie filter—Mechanical filter that removes soft, or low-energy, x-ray beams, minimizing patient exposure and providing a more uniform beam intensity.

cathode-ray tube (CRT)—Monitor used to display CT images.

central processing unit (CPU)—"Brain" of the CT system. The CPU takes information from the data acquisition system and manipulates it so that an image can be formed.

cine imaging—Continuous acquisition scanning without table incrementation.

cluster scanning—Grouping two or more scans into a single breath hold.

contrast resolution—Ability to differentiate small density differences on the image.

convolution—Process of applying a mathematic formula (filter function) to an attenuation profile.

coronal plane—Imaginary plane that divides the body into anterior and posterior sections.

correlate—Display function that allows areas on consecutive cross-sectional images to be traced. Their outline is then superimposed over the scout image.

cupping artifact—Artifact that results from beam hardening. It appears on the image as a vague area of increased density in a somewhat concentric shape around the periphery of an image, similar to the shape of a cup.

data acquisition system—Component of the CT system that samples each detector cell. It is located in the gantry.

detector efficiency—Ability of the detector to capture transmitted photons and change them to electronic signals.

digital audiotape (DAT)—Data storage device that resembles a small cassette tape used for recording music.

display field of view—Determines how much of the raw data are used to display an image. Also called zoom, or target.

dynamic scanning—Process by which scans are acquired quickly, often after a rapid bolus injection of intravenous contrast material.

edge gradient effect—Straight line artifacts that radiate from a high-contrast area, such as bone and soft tissue.

effective slice thickness—Thickness of the slice that is actually represented on the CT image, as opposed to the size selected by the collimator opening. In traditional axial scanning, selected slice thickness is equal to effective slice thickness. However, because of the interpolation process used in spiral scanning, the effective slice thickness may be wider than the selected slice thickness.

equilibrium phase—Last phase of contrast enhancement. Occurs when the attenuation difference between the aorta and the inferior vena cava is less than 10 Hounsfield units.

extravasation—Seepage of intravenous solution into the soft tissue.

floppy disk—Data storage device that may be 5.25 inches in diameter and actually floppy to hold or 3.5 inches in diameter and encased in a firm plastic holder.

geometric efficiency—Space occupied by the detector collimator plates relative to the surface area of the detector.

gray scale—System that assigns a given number of Hounsfield values to each level of gray. The number of Hounsfield values assigned to each level of gray is determined by the window width.

half-scan—Scan produced from a tube arc of less than 360°. Typically acquired from 180° of tube travel, plus the degree of arc from the fan angle. Also called partial scan.

heat capacity—Ability of the system to withstand by-product heat.

heat dissipation—Ability of the system to rid itself of by-product heat.

helical scanning—Scan that consists of a continually rotating x-ray tube with constant x-ray output and uninterrupted table movement. Also called spiral, volumetric, or continuous acquisition scanning.

histogram—Display function that creates a bar graph to show how frequently a range of CT numbers occur within a specified region of interest.

Hounsfield units (HU)—Measure of the beam attenuation capability of a specific structure. Also called pixel values, or CT numbers.

image magnification—Postprocessing method of increasing the image size as it appears on the monitor.

image processor—Component of a CT system that converts digitized data to shades of gray to be displayed on a cathode-ray tube monitor.

image reconstruction—Use of raw data to create a CT image.

ionic/nonionic—Characteristic of intravenous iodinated contrast medium that relates to its chemical composition. The term ionic, when used to describe contrast material, refers to a type that forms ions in a water solution. Nonionic contrast medium does not dissociate and therefore does not ionize in water.

isotonic—Having nearly the same number of particles in solution as water.

kilovolt (kV)—Measure of the high voltage produced by the x-ray generator. Qualitative measure of the x-ray beam.

milliampere (mA)—Measure of the tube current used in the production of x-ray energy. In conjunction with the scan time, it is the quantitative measure of the x-ray beam.

magnetic tape—Data storage device that consists of large reels of tape.

matrix—Grid formed from rows and columns of pixels.

noise—Speckled appearance of the CT image

caused by insufficient photons reaching the detectors.

nonequilibrium phase—Phase of contrast enhancement that follows the bolus phase. It is characterized by a difference of 10 to 30 Hounsfield units between the aorta and the inferior vena cava.

oblique plane—Imaginary plane that is slanted and lies at an angle to one of the three standard planes.

optical disk—Newest type of data storage device. Consists of a disk that resembles a compact disk used to record music. Two types of optical disks are currently available. Those that cannot be erased are referred to as WORM (write once, read many), and those that can be erased and reused are referred to as magnetic optical disks.

osmolality—Structural property of a liquid regarding the number of particles in solution compared with water.

out-of-field artifacts—Streaks, shading, or incorrect Hounsfield numbers that are caused from improper patient positioning.

overscan—Scan produced from 360° of tube travel plus approximately the width of the field of view.

partial scan—Scans produced from a tube arc of less than 360°. Typically acquired from 180° of tube travel, plus the degree of arc from the fan angle. Also called half-scan.

partial volume effect—Process in CT by which different tissue attenuations are averaged to produce one less accurate pixel reading. Also known as volume averaging.

pitch—Relation of table speed to slice thickness.

pixel—Two-dimensional square of data. When arranged in rows and columns, they make up the image matrix.

prospective reconstruction—Image reconstruction process that occurs automatically during a CT scan.

raw data—All measurements obtained from the detector array. Also called scan data.

ray sum—Measurement by the detector of how much the x-ray beam has been attenuated.

referencing the table—Process of manually setting a zero point on the CT table. Generally, this zero point is set at a predetermined anatomic landmark, such as the xiphoid or iliac crest.

reformat—Use of image data to create a view in a different body plane.

region of interest (ROI)—Area on the CT image defined by the operator. The area may be circular, square, elliptic, rectangular, or custom-drawn by the operator. Defining an ROI is the first step in a number of image display and measurement functions.

retrospective reconstruction—Use of raw data to create additional images after the initial examination is completed.

sagittal plane—Imaginary plane that divides the body into right and left sections.

scan data—All measurements obtained from the detector array. Also called raw data.

scan field of view—Area within the gantry for which raw data are acquired. Also called calibration field of view.

scan parameters—Factors that are controlled by the operator and affect the quality of the CT image produced. These factors include milliamperes, kilovolt-peak, scan time, slice thickness, field of view, and algorithm.

scanner generation—Configuration of the x-ray tube to the detector.

slice misregistration—Problem caused when the patient breathes inconsistently between images. It can result in missing areas of anatomy in the CT study.

slip-ring—Mechanism in some CT scanners that allows the x-ray tube to rotate continually in the same direction.

source collimator—Device that resembles small shutters with an opening that adjusts according to the operator's selection of slice thickness. It is located in the x-ray tube and limits the amount of x-ray energy emerging.

spatial resolution—Ability to represent small objects and differentiate between closely spaced objects.

spiral scanning—Continually rotating x-ray tube with constant x-ray output and uninterrupted table movement. Also called helical, volumetric, or continuous acquisition scanning.

view—Complete set of ray sums. Many views are used to produce a single CT image.

volume averaging—Process by which different tissue attenuations are averaged to produce one less accurate pixel reading. Also called partial volume effect.

voxel—Volume element. Cube of data acquired in CT.

window level—Mechanism that selects the center CT value of the window width.

window width—Mechanism that determines the range of Hounsfield numbers that will be represented on a particular image.

z axis—Plane that correlates to the slice thickness, or depth, of a CT slice.

Bibliography

Balfe D, Peterson R, VanDyke J: Normal abdominal and pelvic anatomy. In *Computed Body Tomography with MRI Correlation,* 2nd ed. Edited by Lee J, Sagel S, Stanley R. New York, Raven Press, 1989.

Berland LL: *Practical CT: Technology and Techniques.* New York, Raven Press, 1987.

Bonneville JF, Cattin F, Dietemann JL: In *Computed Tomography of the Pituitary Gland.* Berlin, Springer-Verlag, 1986.

Gado M, Sartor K, Hodges FJ: Spine. In *Computed Body Tomography with MRI Correlation,* 2nd ed. Edited by Lee J, Sagel S, Stanley R. New York, Raven Press, 1989.

General Electric: Fundamentals of Scanning, Broadcast Supplement, 1991.

Glazer H, Balfe D, Sagel S: Neck. In *Computed Body Tomography with MRI Correlation,* 2nd ed. Edited by Lee J, Sagel S, Stanley R. New York, Raven Press, 1989.

Humes D: *Radiocontrast-Induced Nephrotoxicity.* Princeton, NJ, Squibb Diagnostics, 1989.

Image Analysis, Inc.: Promotional material on bone mineral densitometry, 1993.

Katayama H, Yamaguchi K, Kazuka T, et al: Adverse reactions to ionic and nonionic contrast media. *Radiology* 175:621–628, 1990.

Katzberg R: *The Contrast Media Manual.* Baltimore, Williams & Wilkins, 1992.

Lee J, Marx M: Pelvis. In *Computed Body Tomography with MRI Correlation,* 2nd ed. Edited by Lee J, Sagel S, Stanley R. New York, Raven Press, 1989.

Lee SH, Rao K: *Cranial Computed Tomography.* New York, McGraw-Hill, 1983.

Lundsford L: *Modern Stereostactic Neurosurgery.* Boston, Martinus Nijhoff, 1988.

Mancuso A, Hanafee W: *Computed Tomography and Magnetic Resonance Imaging of the Head and Neck.* Baltimore, Williams & Wilkins, 1985.

Murphy WA, Totty WG, Destouer JM, et al: Musculoskeletal system. In *Computed Body Tomography with MRI Correlation,* 2nd ed. Edited by Lee J, Sagel S, Stanley R. New York, Raven Press, 1989.

Palmer FJ: The RACR survey of intravenous contrast media reactions: a preliminary report. *Australian Radiology* 32:8–11, 1988.

Picus D, Weyman PJ, Anderson DJ: Interventional computed tomography. In *Computed Body Tomography with MRI Correlation,* 2nd ed. Edited by Lee J, Sagel S, Stanley R. New York, Raven Press, 1989.

Semba CP, Rubin GD, Dake, MD: Three-dimensional spiral CT angiography of the abdomen. *Semin Ultrasound CT MR* 15(2):133–138, 1994.

Stanley RJ, Koslin DB, Lee JKT: Pancreas. In *Computed Body Tomography with MRI Correlation,* 2nd ed. Edited by Lee J, Sagel S, Stanley R. New York, Raven Press, 1989.

Wang G, Vannier MW: Longitudinal resolution in volumetric x-ray computerized tomography: analytical comparison between conventional and helical computerized tomography. *Med Phys* 21(3):429–431, 1994.

Wilcock KE, Santamaria AB, Frankos VH, et al: Perspectives on adverse reaction rates associated with the use of high osmolar ionic and low osmolar nonionic contrast media. *Journal of the American College of Toxicology* 9(6):563–607, 1990.

Williams A, Haugton V: *Cranial Computed Tomography: A Comprehensive Text.* St. Louis, Mosby, 1985.

Index

Note: Page numbers in *italics* denote illustrations; those followed by (t) denote tables.

A

Abdomen, scanning protocol for, 81-84, 82(t), 83(t)
Abscess drainage, CT for, 96, 97
  supplies for, 97(t)
Adrenals, scanning protocol for, 83, 83(t)
Algorithm, image quality and, 22
Allergies, patient history of, 64
Anatomic position, 60, *61*
Angiography, hepatic CT, 56
  radiation dose from, 46
  three-dimensional spiral CT, 92-94, *93*
Annotations, image, 36, 62, 63
Anterior, definition of, 60
Archiving methods, 65
Artifacts, beam hardening, 11, *11*
  image quality and, 22
  out-of-field, 16
  troubleshooting for, 23(t)
Attenuation, beam, 5-7
Attenuation profile, 13, 15
Auditory scanning protocol, 74(t)
Axial plane, changing imaging plane to, 60, 61
  definition of, 60
Axial slices, 26, *26*

B

Back projection, 15
Barium sulfate solutions, for bowel opacification, 56-57
Biopsy, CT-guided, 96-97
  supplies for, 97(t)
Biphasic injection, of contrast media, 56
Blood-brain barrier, and seizures from contrast media, 52-53
Bolus injection, of contrast media, 56
Bolus phase, of tissue enhancement, 55
Bone densitometry, 91, *92*
Brachial plexus, scanning protocol for, 78(t)
Brain metastasis, seizures with, from contrast media, 52-53
Brain scanning protocols, 71, 71(t), *72*, 76
  for pituitary and sella turcica, 71, *73-74*, 73(t), 76
  for posterior fossa and skull base, 71, 72(t)
  window width for, 33-34
Breathing instructions, for scanning, 63

C

Caudal, definition of, 60
Centigray, 43
Chest, scanning protocol for, 79-80, 79(t), *80*, 80(t)
Cine imaging, 31
Collimation, 12
  radiation dose and, 48
Consent forms, for use of contrast media, 65

Contiguous scans, 63
Contrast media, for abdominal scanning, 81-82, 83
  annotation of, 63
  beam attenuation and, 5-6, *5*
  for brain scanning, 71
  for chest scanning, 79-80
  consent for use of, 65
  gastrointestinal, barium sulfate solutions as, 56-57
    water-soluble agents as, 57
  intravascular, administration of, 55
    central nervous system involvement and, 52-53
    effects of, on tissue enhancement, 55
    extravasation of, 54-55
    high-osmolality vs. low-osmolality, 53, 53(t)
    injection methods for, 55-56
    injection route for, 53-54
    ionic vs. nonionic, 51-52
    osmolality of, 51-52
    renal clearance of, 52, 52(t)
    viscosity of, 51
  for musculoskeletal system scanning, 90
  for pelvic scanning, 85
  protocols for, 69
  for repeat scans, 63
  for spine scanning, 86, 88-89
  spiral scanning and, 31
Contrast resolution, 12
Convolution, 15, 22
Coronal plane, changing imaging plane to, 60, 61
  definition of, 60
Correlate function, 37, *38*
Cranial, definition of, 60
CT dose index (CTDI), 43
CT numbers, 6, *6*
Cursor measurement, of Hounsfield units, 35

D

Data, raw vs. image, in image reconstruction, 15
Data acquisition, and CT image creation, 8-13
  methods of, cine imaging as, 31
    continuous acquisition scanning as, 26-31
    standard axial acquisition scanning as, 24-26
Density, beam attenuation and, 5
Dental scanning, 91, *93*
Detectors, configuration of, 8
  efficiency of, radiation dose and, 48
  optimal characteristics of, 12
  scatter acceptance and, 13, *14*
  solid-state crystal, 12, 12(t), 13
  xenon gas, 12-13, 12(t)
Digital audiotape (DAT), for archiving, 65
Directional instructions, input of, 62
Disks, for archiving, 65

Display functions, advanced, correlate, 37, *38*
   histogram, 36, *37*
   pixel value, 36–37
   reformation, 37–38, *39*, 40
Distal, definition of, 60
Distance measurements, image display and, 36
Dorsal, definition of, 60
Double dose delay, 71
Double window setting, 34
Drip infusion, of contrast media, 55–56
Dual window setting, 34
Dynamic sequential bolus CT, 56

E
Electron beam imaging, 9
Enhancement techniques, *see also* Contrast media
   with gastrointestinal contrast materials, 56–57
   with intravascular contrast materials, 51–56
Equilibrium phase, of tissue enhancement, 55, 81
Exposures, typical number of, in CT, 9, 10(t)
Extravasation, of contrast media, 54–55

F
Facial bone, scanning protocol for, 75(t)
Feed, 13
Field of view, calibration, 15
   display, 16–17, *17*
   image quality and, 21–22
   radiation dose and, 48
   scan, 15–16, *16*
Filming techniques, 65, *66*
Filtering, for artifact reduction, 11, *12*, 15
Filters, bow tie, 11
   reconstruction, radiation dose and, 49
Filtration, radiation dose and, 47–48
Fluoroscopy, radiation dose from, 46
Fossa, posterior, scanning protocol for, 72(t)

G
Gantry, continuous rotation, 21
   and CT image creation, 9
Generator, and CT image creation, 9
Gray (Gy), 43
Gray scale, image display and, 33

H
Half-scans, 20
Hard copy, 65
Head, coronal scanning position for, 61–62
   scanning protocols for, 74(t), 75(t), *76*
Heat capacity, of x-ray tube, 8
Heat dissipation, with spiral scanning, 30–31
   of x-ray tube, 8
Hemangiomas, liver, dynamic scanning of, 25
Histogram, 36, *37*
History, patient, 64–65
Horizontal plane, definition of, 60
Hounsfield units, 6, *6*
   and standard deviation, 35–36
   window settings and, 33–34

I
Image creation, data acquisition for, 8–13
   image reconstruction and, 13, 15–17
Image display, advanced functions for, 36–40
   distance measurements and, 36
   Hounsfield measurements and, 35–36

image annotation for, 36
image magnification for, 34–35
multiple, 36
priority reconstruction and, 36
reference image and, 36
window settings for, 33–34
Image quality, factors affecting, algorithm, 22
   artifacts, 22
   field of view, 21–22
   kilovolt-peak setting, 21
   milliampere-second setting, 19–20
   scan time, 20–21
   slice thickness, 21
   tube arc, 20
Imaging planes, 60–62, *62*, *63*
Incrementation, 13
Index, 13
Inferior, definition of, 60
Injection, of contrast media, 53–54, 55–56
Interpolation, software, 28
Interventional computed tomography, 96–97

K
Kidneys, in excretion of contrast media, 52
   failure of, from contrast media, 52, 52(t)
   patient history of function of, 64
   scanning protocol for, 83–84, 83(t)
Kilovolt-peak setting, image quality and, 19, 21
   radiation dose and, 47

L
Larynx, scanning protocol for, 77(t)
Lateral, definition of, 60
Localization scans, radiation dose from, 48–49
Longitudinal plane, definition of, 60

M
mA, radiation dose and, 47
Magnetic tape, for archiving, 65
Magnification, image, 34–35
Matrix, 4
   size of, and radiation dose, 48
Mechanical flow-control injectors, for injection of
   contrast media, 54
Medial, definition of, 60
Median plane, definition of, 60
Midsagittal plane, definition of, 60
Milliampere seconds, 19
Milliampere-second setting, image quality and, 19–20
   in spiral scanning, 30
Motion, spiral scanning and, 31
Multiple scan average dose (MSAD), 43
Musculoskeletal system, scanning protocol for, 90,
   90(t)

N
Neck, scanning protocol for, 77, 77(t), 78(t)
Noise, image quality and, 49
Nonequilibrium phase, of tissue enhancement, 55

O
Oblique planes, definition of, 60, *62*
Optical disks, for archiving, 65
Orbit, scanning protocol for, 75(t)
Osmolality, of contrast media, side effects from,
   51–52, 53, 53(t)
Overscan, 20

P

Pancreas, scanning protocol for, 82–83, 83(t)
Parasagittal plane, definition of, 60
Partial volume effect, 7, 21
Patient size, radiation dose and, 48
Pelvis, scanning protocol for, 85, 85(t)
Peritonitis, barium, 57
Pitch, radiation dose and, 48
    in spiral scanning, 29–30, *29*
Pituitary gland, scanning protocol for, 71, *73–74*,
        73(t), 76
Pixel, 4, 5, *5*
    determining size of, 17
Pixel value function, 36–37
Planes, imaging, *see* Imaging planes *and specific*
        planes
Portography, CT, 56
Position, patient, for imaging in different planes,
        60–62
Posterior, definition of, 60
Proximal, definition of, 60

Q

Quality factor (Q), 43
Quantum mottle, 49
Quantum noise, 49

R

Rad, 43
Radiation, ionizing, 43
    scatter, collimation and, 12
        detector arrangement and, 13, *14*
Radiation dose, to patient, 43–46, *44, 45, 46*
    factors affecting, 46–49
    relationship of, to image quality, 49
    slice spacing and, 63–64
    slice thickness and, 7, 63–64
Radiation equivalent man (rem), 43
Radiography, conventional, radiation dose from, 44,
        45–46
    interventional, radiation dose from, 46
Rapid scan, 25
Ray, 13
Ray sum, 13
Reconstruction of images, 13, 15–17
    priority, 36
    prospective, 15
    retrospective, 15
Reference image function, 36
Reformation, multiplanar, 37–38, *39*
    real-time, 37
    three-dimensional, 38, 40
Region of interest (ROI), 35
Rem (radiation equivalent man), 43
Renal excretion, of contrast media, 52
Renal failure, from contrast media, 52, 52(t)
Renal function, patient history of, 64
Repeat scans, radiation dose from, 48
Roentgen (R), 43
Rotation angle, radiation dose and, 47

S

Sagittal plane, definition of, 60
Scan field diameter, radiation dose and, 48
Scanners, design of, 8
    generation of, 9, *10*
        radiation dose and, 46–47

manufacturers of, 3
    pipeline, 24
Scanning methods, cine imaging, 31
    cluster scanning, 25–26
    continuous acquisition scanning, 3, 26–31, *26*
    dynamic scanning, 24–25
    helical scanning, 3, 26–31, *26*
    nonincremental scanning, 25
    rapid acquisition scanning, 25
    spiral scanning, 3, 26–31, *26*
        injection techniques for, 56
        radiation dose from, 48
    standard axial acquisition scanning, 24–26
Scanning parameters, image quality and, 19–22
Scanning procedures, routine, 62–64
Scanning protocols, for abdomen, 81–84
    for chest, 79–80
    for head and brain, 71–76
    for musculoskeletal system, 90
    for neck, 77–78
    for pelvis, 85
    for spine, 86–89
Scan time, with cluster scanning, 25–26
    image quality and, 20–21
    with spiral scanning, 31
Scout image, 62, 63
Seizures, from contrast media, 52–53
Sella turcica, scanning protocol for, 73(t), 76
Sievert (Sv), 43
Sinuses, coronal vs. axial imaging of, 61, *64*
    scanning protocol for, 75(t), 76
Skull base, scanning protocol for, 71, 72(t)
Slice, elements of, 4, *4*
Slice misregistration, 24, *25*
    spiral scanning and, 31
Slice spacing, radiation dose and, 48, 63–64
Slice thickness, image quality and, 21
    radiation dose and, 48, 63–64
    in spiral scanning, 27–29, *28, 29*
Slip-ring scanners, reduced scan time with, 20–21
Source collimator, 12
Spatial resolution, 19
Spine, scanning protocol for, 86, 86(t), *87*, 87(t),
        88–89, *88, 89*
Standard deviation, Hounsfield units and, 35–36
Step, 13
Stereotactic surgical planning, *94*, 94–95
Superior, definition of, 60

T

Table, patient, 13
Target, 16
Temporomandibular joint, scanning protocol for, 75(t)
Transverse plane, definition of, 60
Tube arc, image quality and, 20

V

Ventral, definition of, 60
Vertical plane, definition of, 60
View, 13
Viscosity, of contrast media, side effects from, 51
Volume averaging, 7, 21
Voxel, 4

W

Water-soluble solutions, for bowel opacification, 57
Window settings, image display and, 33–34, *34*

Write once, read many (WORM) disks, for archiving, 65

X
X-ray beam, attenuation of, 5–7
    sources of, 9–11
X-ray radiation, 43
X-ray tube, detector and, 8
    heat capacity of, 10

heat dissipation rate of, 10
stress on, 9–10

Z
Z axis, 4, 4
Zoom, 16